CW00520319

KETO DIET

FOR WOMEN AFTER 50

Enjoy the Perfect Meal Plan, Ideal Also For Vegetarians, With Simple and Fast Ketogenic Recipes to Boost Weight Loss and Increase Your Energy While Reducing Menopause Symptoms

---

Tess Connors

© Copyright 2021 – All rights reserved.

The content contained within this book may not be reproduced, duplicated or transmitted without direct written permission from the author or the publisher.

Under no circumstances will any blame or legal responsibility be held against the publisher, or author, for any damages, reparation, or monetary loss due to the information contained within this book. Either directly or indirectly.

Legal Notice:

This book is copyright protected. This book is only for personal use. You cannot amend, distribute, sell, use, quote or paraphrase any part, or the content within this book, without the consent of the author or publisher.

Disclaimer Notice:

Please note the information contained within this document is for educational and entertainment purposes only. All effort has been executed to present accurate, up to date, and reliable, complete information. No warranties of any kind are declared or implied. Readers acknowledge that the author is not engaging in the rendering of legal, financial, medical or professional advice. The content within this book has been derived from various sources. Please consult a licensed professional before attempting any techniques outlined in this book.

By reading this document, the reader agrees that under no circumstances is the author responsible for any losses, direct or indirect, which are incurred as a result of the use of information contained within this document, including, but not limited to, — errors, omissions, or inaccuracies.

Table of Contents:

INTRODUCTION

The health benefits of the Keto diet are not different for men or women, but the speed at which they are reached does differ. As mentioned, women's bodies are a lot other when it comes to burning fats and losing weight. For example, by design, women have at least 10% more body fat than men. No matter how fit you are, this is just an aspect of being a woman you must consider. Don't be hard on yourself if you notice that it seems like men can lose weight easier — that's because they can! What women have in additional body fat, men typically have the same in muscle mass. This is why men tend to see faster external results because that added muscle mass means that their metabolism rates are higher. That increased metabolism means that fat and energy get burned more quickly. When you are on Keto, though, the internal change is happening right away.

Your metabolism is unique, but it will also be slower than a man's by nature. Since muscle can burn more Cal. than fat, the weight seems to fall off of men, giving them the ability to reach the opportunity for muscle growth quickly. This should not be something that holds you back from starting your Keto journey. As long as you keep these realistic bodily factors in mind, you won't be left wondering why it takes you a little longer to start losing weight. This point will come for you, but it will take a little bit more of a process that you must be committed to following through with.

A woman can experience another unique condition, but a man cannot be PCOS or Polycystic Ovary Syndrome, a hormonal imbalance that causes cysts' development. These cysts can cause pain, interfere with normal reproductive function, and burst in extreme and dangerous cases. PCOS is ubiquitous among women, affecting up to 10% of the entire female population. Surprisingly, most women are not even aware that they have the condition. Around 70% of women have PCOS, which is undiagnosed. This condition can cause a significant hormonal imbalance, therefore affecting your metabolism. It can also inevitably lead to weight gain, making it even harder to see results while following diet plans. To stay on top of your health, you must make sure that you are going to the gynecologist regularly.

Menopause is another reality that must be faced by women, especially as we age. Most women begin the process of menopause in their mid-40s. Men do not go through menopause, so they are spared from another condition that causes slower metabolism and weight gain. When you start menopause, it is easy to gain weight and lose muscle. Once menopause begins, most women lose power at a much faster rate and conversely gain weight, despite dieting and exercise regimens. Keto can, therefore, be the right diet plan for you. Regardless of what your body is doing naturally, via processes like menopause, your internal systems are still going to be making the switch from running on carbs to deriving energy from fats.

CHAPTER 1: What Are The Advantages And Disadvantages Of Keto Dieting?

The Keto dieting has been proven to have many advantages for people over 50. Here are some of the best.

Strengthens bones

When people get older, their bones weaken. At 50, your bones at likely not as strong as they used to be; however, you can keep them in excellent conditions. Consuming milk to give calcium cannot do enough to strengthen your bones. What you can do is to make use of the Keto diet as it is low in toxins. Toxins negatively affect the absorption of nutrients, and so with this, your bones can take in all they need.

Eradicates inflammation

Few things are worse than the pain from an inflamed joint or muscle. Arthritis, for instance, can be tough to bear. When you use the ketosis diet, the production of cytokines would be reduced. Cytokines inflammation and so, their eradication would reduce it.

It eradicates nutrients deficiency.

Keto focuses on consuming precisely what you need. If you use a great Keto plan, your body will lack no nutrients and will not suffer any deficiency.

Reduced hunger

The reason we find it hard to stick to diets is hunger. It doesn't matter your age. Diets do not become more comfortable to stick to. We may have a mental picture of the healthy body we want. We may even have clear visuals of the kind of life we want to leave once free from unhealthy living but none of that matters when hunger enters the scene. However, the Keto diet is a diet that combats this problem. Keto diet focuses on consuming plenty of Prot.. Prot. are filling and do not let you feel hungry too quickly. Also, when your carb levels are reduced, your appetite takes a hit. It is a win-win situation.

Weight loss

Keto not only burns fat, but it also reduces that crave for food. Combined, these are two great ways to lose weight. It is one of the diets that has proven to help the most in weight loss. The Keto diet has been proven to be one of the best ways to burn stubborn belly fat while keeping yourself revitalized and healthy.

Reduces blood sugar and insulin

After 50, monitoring blood sugar can be a real struggle. Cutting down on cars drastically reduces both insulin levels and blood sugar levels. This means that the Keto diet will benefit millions as many people struggle with insulin complications and high blood sugar levels. It has been proven to help when some people embark on Keto, and they cut up to half of the carbs they consume. It's a treasure for those with diabetes and insulin resistance. A study was carried out on people with type 2 diabetes. After cutting down on carbs, within six months, 95 percent of the people could reduce or stop using their glucose-lowering medication.

Lower levels of triglycerides

A lot of people do not know what triglycerides are. Triglycerides are molecules of fat in your blood. They are known to circulate in the bloodstream and can be very dangerous. High levels of triglycerides can cause heart failures and heart diseases. However, Keto is known to reduce these levels.

Reduces acne

Although young people mostly suffer acne, there are cases of people above 50 having it. Moreover, Keto is not only for persons after 50. Acne is not only caused by blocked pores. There are quite several things proven to drive it. One of these things is your blood sugar. When you consume processed and refined carbs, it affects gut bacteria and results in blood sugar levels fluctuation. When the gut bacteria and sugar levels are affected, the skin suffers. However, when you embark on the Keto diet, you cut off on carbs intake, which means that in the very first place, your gut bacteria will not be affected, thereby cutting off that avenue to develop.

Increases HDL levels

HDL refers to high-density lipoprotein. When your HDL levels are compared to your LDL levels and are not found low, your risk of developing heart disease is lowered. This is great for persons over 50 as heart diseases suddenly become more probable. Eating fats and reducing your intake of Carbs is one of the most secure ways to increase your high-density lipoprotein levels.

Reduces LDL levels

High levels of LDL can be very problematic when you attain 50. This is because LDL refers to bad cholesterol. People with high levels of this cholesterol are more likely to get heart attacks. When you reduce the number of carbs you consume, you will increase lousy LDL particles'

size. However, this will reduce the total LDL particles as they would have increased in size. Smaller LDL particles have been linked to heart diseases, while larger ones have been proven to have lower risks attached.

May help combat cancer

I termed this under 'may' because research on this is not as extensive and conclusive as we would like it to be. However, there is proof of supporting it. Firstly, it helps reduce the levels of blood sugar, which lowers insulin complications, reducing the risk of developing cancers related to insulin levels. Also, Keto places more oxidative stress on cancer cells than normal cells, thereby making it great for chemotherapy. After fifty, the risk of developing cancer is still existent, and so, Keto is a lifesaver.

May lower blood pressure

High blood pressure plagues adults much more than it does young ones. Once you attain 50, you must monitor your blood pressure rates. Reduction in the intake of Carbs is a proven way to lower your blood pressure. When you cut down on your carbs and lower your blood sugar levels, you significantly reduce your chances of getting other diseases.

Combats metabolic syndrome

As you grow older, you may find that you struggle to control your blood sugar level.

Metabolic syndrome is another condition that has been proven to influence diabetes and heart disease development. The symptoms associated with metabolic syndrome include but are not limited to high triglycerides, obesity, high blood sugar level, and low levels of high-density lipoprotein cholesterol.

However, you will find that reducing your level of carbohydrate intake dramatically affects this. You will improve your health and majorly attack all the above-listed symptoms. Keto diet helps to fight against metabolic syndrome, which is a big win.

Great for the heart

People over the age of 50 have been proven to have more chances of developing heart diseases. Keto diet has been proven to be great for the heart.

As it increases acceptable cholesterol levels and reduces harmful cholesterol levels, you will find that partaking in the Keto diet proves exceptionally beneficial for your health.

May reduce seizure risks

When you change your intake levels, the combination of protein, fat, and carbs, as we explained before, your body will go into ketosis. Ketosis has been proven to reduce seizure levels in people who have epilepsy.

When they do not respond to treatment, the ketosis treatment is used. This has been done for decades.

Combats brain disorders

Keto doesn't end there. It also combats Alzheimer's and Parkinson's disease. Some parts of your brain can only burn glucose, and so, your body needs it. If you do not consume carbs, your lover will make use of protein to produce glucose.

Your brain can also burn ketones. Ketones are formed when your carb level is deficient. With this, the ketogenic diet has been used f r plenty of years to treat epilepsy in children who aren't responding to drugs. For adults, it can work the same magic as it is now being linked to treating Alzheimer's and Parkinson's disease

Helps women suffering from the polycystic ovarian syndrome

This syndrome affects women of all ages. PCOS is short for the polycystic ovarian syndrome. The polycystic ovarian syndrome is an endocrine disorder that results in enlarged ovaries with cysts. These cysts are dangerous and cause other complications. It has been proven that a high intake of Carbs negatively affects women suffering from the polycystic ovarian syndrome. When a woman with PCOS cuts down on carbs and embarks on the Keto diet, the polycystic ovarian syndrome falls under attack.

It is beyond doubt that the Keto diet is beneficial in so many ways that it almost looks unreal. If you are to embark on the Keto diet, there are several things you must know.

Disadvantages

Your body will have an adjustment period. It depends from person to person on how many days that will be, but when you start any new diet or exercise routine, your body has to adjust to the new normal. With the keto diet, you are drastically cutting your Carbs intake, so the body must adapt.

You may feel slow, weak, exhausted, and like you are not thinking as quick or fast as you used to. It just means your body is adjusting to keto, and once this adjustment period is done, you will see the weight loss results you anticipated.

If you are an athlete, you may need more Carbs. If you still want to try keto as an athlete, you must talk to your Nutritionist or trainer to see how the diet can be tweaked for you. Most athletes require a greater intake of carbs than the keto diet requires, which means they may have to up their information to ensure they have the energy for their training sessions.

High endurance sports (like rugby or soccer) and heavy weightlifting require a greater intake of Carbs. If you're an athlete wanting to follow keto and gain the health benefits, it's essential you first talk to your trainer before making any changes to your diet.

You have to count your daily macros carefully! This can be tough for beginners, and even people already on keto can become lazy about this. People are often used to eating what they want without worrying about just how many g of protein or carbs it contains. With keto, you have to be meticulous about counting your intake to ensure you are maintaining the necessary keto breakdown (75% fat, 20% protein, ~5% carbs). The closer you stick to this, the better results you will see regarding weight loss and other health benefits.

If your weight loss has stalled or you're not feeling as energetic as you hoped, it could be because your macros are off. Find a free calorie counting app that and be sure you look at the ingredients of everything you're eating and cooking.

CHAPTER 2: How to Manage Yourself during a Keto Diet

The Keto Diet Mindset

Like any other life-transforming endeavor, the keto diet regimen is dependent on your mindset. You must be prepared to face the emotional, physical, and psychological obstacles that will arise in the course of achieving your goals. This underpins the impact the diet will have on your life. One of the fundamental elements of keto is a mindset that is equipped to deal with many obstacles and challenges.

For some, the desire to lose weight is the underlying impetus, while others are motivated by living healthier lives. In some cases, a person may be forced to consider a diet change for medical or biological reasons. Regardless of the motivation, maintaining the right mindset always determines the success of a change in diet. In this regard, attaining an appropriate attitude is the first step towards initiating and benefitting from a keto-based diet.

The Right Mindset for a Keto Diet

When beginning a keto diet, the first phase of your journey must be adopting an appropriate mindset that will allow you to make this lifestyle change successfully. While you might set your goals right from the start, you must consider that your energy and enthusiasm is likely to wane over time. For most people, this results in failure, which is then translated into frustration and the loss of confidence in the ketogenic diet. By emotionally and psychologically preparing oneself for the journey ahead, achieving this feat quite quickly is possible.

You must first acknowledge and accept in your mind that the diet does work and that you can experience its impact on your life. This is the first and most crucial thought process to actively and judiciously stick to the plan. If you have tried other diet plans in the past with little success, this particular thought process may be hard to come by. However, by shifting your focus to scientific and factual material regarding the diet, you may begin to appreciate its efficacy.

The capacity to individually internalize this concept forms the basis of the essential mindset for a keto diet. By eliminating any form of doubt in your mind concerning the benefits and impact of a keto diet, you set yourself up for success. This is because it helps you stay focused on the outcome while ignoring the day to day challenges and distractions that will undoubtedly arise. Internalization and appreciation of the benefits and effectiveness of the keto diet create the necessary momentum needed to consistently adhere to the stipulations that come with implementing the diet.

The elimination of excuses is also fundamental if you are to realize the benefits of a keto diet. For most people, dietary changes are seen as significant transformations that occur overnight. For a woman in her 50s, this can prove daunting and even scary. When you have already lived on a different diet for half a century, you have an internal block that causes you to doubt your ability to change your diet's content. You are likely to develop numerous excuses and justifications as to why such a diet may not work for you. If you are looking at a keto diet as a total overhaul of how you are a person, then there is a higher likelihood you will find the endeavor too arduous even to try.

By holding onto the notion, a keto diet is only successful when drastic and dramatic changes are made in your life. You save yourself back with your thoughts. In most cases, this line of thinking should raise the red flag of fear and unnecessary excuses. While your former attempts at dieting may have informed such notions, you must approach a keto diet with a fresh and curious mind.

It is also essential to approach the keto diet as a new partner that will bring you much-awaited love, compassion, and care. In this case, therefore, you must assume a sense of self-love and care to ensure that it works. Day-to-day interactions and experiences can often impose a sense of negativity and self-loathing. In failing to accomplish various goals, meet specific demands, or achieve individual personal, professional, or social goals, the burden of guilt and self-hate is likely to emerge.

Such a state of mind is limited in numerous ways, and as such, it cannot achieve the desired frequency of caring for itself. Once you learn to be kind and patient with yourself, you realize life has its ups and downs. Regardless of these challenges, you must give yourself the time and space to fail, learn, and grow as you go. The self-care mindset is crucial for effectiveness on the keto diet. By appreciating and loving yourself, you initiate a process in which your well-being is paramount to your survival. As such, you are ready to undertake any efforts whatsoever to improve the quality of your life. A sense of purpose and limitlessness becomes a constant aspect of your life, and as such, you can see your goals and ambitions through.

As is the case, with newest things, encounters, and experiences, you are likely to continuously feel the need to remind yourself of the feeling continually. For instance, when you buy a new phone, you may not want to put it down even as you explore its features and quirks. Over time your adoration for the new item may turn into an obsession or compulsive behavior that can be hard to break. The same analogy works when it comes to dieting. In setting out to try a new diet, as is the case with a keto diet, you may fixate on the expected outcomes and results. It is essential to note the fact that while your weight may be slow to change, there is a likelihood your muscle structure will have a change in terms of getting leaner.

By moving away from the metric-tracking mentality, you allow yourself the time to acclimate to the diet and notice the overall changes it brings about in your physical, psychological, and emotional well-being rather than fixating on the pounds lost or gained.

Cognitively preparing for the long-haul is also vital in achieving the goals and benefits of a keto diet.

The best way to appreciate a ketogenic diet is by looking at it as a lifestyle change rather than a change in dietary intakes. While the benefits of the diet are factual and well documented, they take time to come about. However, most people believe that a keto diet is a quick fix solution that allows them to transform their health, weight, and body shape within weeks or months. Having gleaned information from various media platforms such individuals are quick to adopt the diet with the hope of having an overnight transformation.

The quick-fix mindset is one of the surest ways of failing in your pursuit to experience the benefits of a ketogenic diet. You must be willing to endure for the long-term goals while celebrating the short-term gains. A two-week on a two-month keto diet may accord you the much need for weight loss. However, such changes are likely to disappear just as fast in the absence of long-term commitment.

Strategies to Develop the Right Mindset for a Keto Diet

Having understood the dynamics surrounding the perfect keto diet mindset, you may wonder how you will achieve such a feat. In other words, you want to establish the actual and practical steps towards developing a paradigm shift. The fields of psychology and behavioral science have been instrumental in expanding knowledge and information surrounding human behavior.

Being aware of your Inner and Outer Surrounding

In this regard, the first and most important strategy is raising awareness of both inner and outer surroundings. With food as a crucial trigger of behavior and habit, maintaining a sense of awareness regarding your thought patterns, cravings, and moment-to-moment activities offers the first step towards mastering your dietary behavior.

To build upon your awareness, you might need to keep a journal as one way of keeping track of your thought patterns and activities. With this in place, it becomes easier to review your day while noticing recurrent thoughts and actions. This will prove crucial in helping you plan your day concerning meals and exercises while keeping track of your dietary intake. Most importantly, however, it will help you cultivate the discipline needed concerning keeping track of your consumption patterns.

Keeping an Open Mind

With your awareness in check, you will need to strive to have an open mind considering the keto diet's mixed results from one person to another. To establish a keto-diet mindset, it will be imperative that you remain as accessible as possible to new ideas, experiments, lessons, disappointments, and victories. Having a fixed mindset regarding the outcomes and expectations from a keto diet serves no purpose at all. You should not approach a keto diet experience with pre-established ideas and notions.

The Willingness to put in the work

While most media depictions of keto diets revolve around quick and short-term gains associated with the change, the reality is far more arduous and lengthy. Beyond the glamour of abs, swift loss of weight, and bright and glowing skin, you must be willing to invest your time and resources to realize your health and diet goals.

This translates to creating time to educate yourself and gain the knowledge and skills necessary to actualize your keto diet dream.

The readiness to make Changes in Your Life

The attainment of a keto diet mindset is also contingent upon your ability to make changes across various areas of your life. Having appreciated the food and eating as habitual behaviors, you must be able to overcome and transform multiple aspects of your life if you enjoy the benefits of a keto diet. This requires a comprehensive audit of your life with a focus on your habits and behavior over time. Your ability to change primarily lies in your comprehension of the factors around your day-to-day life.

As your work towards achieving your healthy diet goal, the need for change will arise from every other corner. Any form of resistance from any faculty of your life may result in unprecedented outcomes concerning your dieting. In essence, in committing to a keto diet, you must be ready to endure various uncomfortable experiences in the short-term.

Visualization

Visualization entails creating mental images of yourself in a healthier, leaner, and more confident state. This means taking time to capture all the upsides that will result from your efforts to transform yourself. You will need to look at the type of relationships you will have, the health benefits associated with the changes you make, and, most importantly, what it will take for you to achieve your goals.

CHAPTER 3: Ketogenic Diet Can Aid With the Signs and Symptoms of Aging and Menopause

For aging women, menopause will bring severe changes and challenges, but the ketogenic diet can help you switch gears effortlessly to continue enjoying a healthy and happy life. Menopause can upset hormonal levels in women, which consequently affects brainpower and cognitive abilities. Furthermore, due to fewer estrogens and progesterone production, your sex drive declines, and you suffer from sleep issues and mood problems. Let's have a look at how a ketogenic diet will help solve these side effects.

Enhanced Cognitive Functions

Usually, the hormone estrogen ensures the continuous flow of glucose into your brain. But after menopause, the estrogen levels begin to drop dramatically, so does the amount of glucose reaching the bran. As a result, your available brainpower will start to deteriorate. However, by following the keto diet for women over 50, glucose intake is circumvented. This results in enhanced cognitive functions and brain activity.

Hormonal Balance

Usually, women face significant symptoms of menopause due to hormonal imbalances. The keto diet for women over 50 works by stabilizing these imbalances such as estrogen—this aids in experiencing fewer and bearable menopausal symptoms like hot flashes. The keto diet also balances blood sugar levels and insulin and helps in controlling insulin sensitivity.

Intensified Sex Drive

The keto diet surges the absorption of vitamin D, which is essential for enhancing sex drive. Vitamin D ensures stable testosterone levels and other sex hormones that could become unstable due to low levels of testosterone.

Better Sleep

Glucose disturbs your blood sugar levels dramatically, which in turn leads to a low quality of sleep. Along with other menopausal symptoms, good sleep becomes a massive problem as you age. The keto diet for women over 50 not only balances blood glucose levels but also stabilizes other hormones like cortisol, melatonin, and serotonin, warranting an improved and better sleep.

Reduces inflammation

Menopause can upsurge the inflammation levels by letting potential harmful invaders in our system, which result in uncomfortable and painful symptoms. Keto diet for women over 50 uses healthy anti-inflammatory fats to reduce inflammation and lower pain in your joints and bones.

Fuel your brain

Are you aware that your brain is composed of 60% fat or more? This infers that it needs an enormous amount of fat to keep it functioning optimally. In other words, the ketones from the keto diet serve as the energy source that fuels your brain cells.

Nutrient deficiencies

Aging women tend to have higher deficiencies in essential nutrients such as an iron deficiency, which leads to brain fog and fatigue—Vitamin B12 deficiency, which leads to neurological conditions like Dementia. Fats deficiency can lead to problems with cognition, skin, vision, and Vitamin D deficiency that cause cognitive impairment in older adults, increase the risk of heart disease and contribute to developing cancer. On a keto diet, the high-quality Prot. ensure adequate and excellent sources of these essential nutrients.

Controlling Blood Sugar

Research has suggested a link between insufficient blood sugar levels and brain diseases such as Alzheimer's disease, Parkinson's Disease, or Dementia. Some factors contributing to Alzheimer's disease may include:

- Enormous intake of Carbs, especially from fructose—which is drastically reduced in the ketogenic diet.

- Lack of nutritional fats and good cholesterol — which are copious and healthy in the keto diet

Keto diet helps control blood sugar and improve nutrition, which in turn improves insulin response and resistance and protects against memory loss, which is often a part of aging.

CHAPTER 4: Useful and Harmful Foods to Do Well On a Keto Diet

I've had people complain about the difficulty of switching their grocery list to one that's Ketogenic-friendly. The fact is that food is expensive, and most of the food you have in your fridge is probably packed full of Carbs. It is why if you're committing to a Ketogenic Diet, you need to do a clean sweep. That's right, everything that's packed with Carbs should be identified and set aside to make sure that you are not overeating.

WHAT TO EAT
ON THE KETO DIET?

Fats and Oils

Because fats will be included as part of all your meals, we recommend choosing the highest quality ingredients you can afford. Some of your best choices for fat are:

- Ghee or Clarified butter
- Avocado
- Coconut Oil
- Red Palm Oil
- Butter
- Coconut Butter
- Peanut Butter
- Chicken Fat
- Beef Tallow
- Non-hydrogenated Lard
- Macadamias and other nuts
- Egg Yolks
- Fish rich in Omega-3 Fatty Acids: salmon, mackerel, trout, tuna, and shellfish

Protein

Those on a keto diet will generally keep fat intake high, carbohydrate intake low, and protein intake at a moderate level. Some on the keto diet for weight loss have better success with higher protein and lower fat intake.

- Fresh meat: beef, veal, lamb, chicken, duck, pheasant, pork, etc.
- Deli meats: bacon, sausage, ham (make sure to watch out for added sugar and other fillers)
- Eggs: preferably free-range or organic eggs
- Fish: wild-caught salmon, catfish, halibut, trout, tuna, etc.
- Other seafood: lobster, crab, oyster, clams, mussels, etc.
- Peanut Butter: this is an excellent source of protein, but make sure to choose a brand that contains no added sugar

Dairy

Compared to other weight-loss diets, the keto diet encourages you to choose dairy products that are full fat. Some of the best dairy products that you can choose are:

- Hard and soft cheese: cream cheese, mozzarella, cheddar, etc.
- Cottage cheese
- Heavy whipping cream
- Sour cream
- Full-fat yogurt

Vegetables

Overall, vegetables are rich in vitamin and minerals that contribute to a healthy body. However, if you're aiming to avoid carbs, you should limit starchy vegetables such as potatoes, yams, peas, corn, beans, and most legumes.

Other vegetables that are high in Carbs, such as parsnips and squash, should also be limited. Instead, stick with green leafy vegetables and other low-carb veggies. Choose local or organic varieties if it fits with your budget.

- Spinach
- Lettuce
- Collard greens
- Mustard greens
- Bok choy
- Kale
- Alfalfa sprouts
- Celery
- Tomato
- Broccoli
- Cauliflower

Fruits

Your choice of fruit on the keto diet is typically restricted to avocado and berries because fruits are high in Carbs and sugar.

Drinks

- Water
- Black coffee
- Herbal tea
- Wine: white wine and dry red wine are OK if they are only consumed occasionally.

Others

- Homemade mayo: if you want to buy mayo from the store, make sure that you watch out for added sugar
- Homemade mustard
- Any spices or herbs
- Stevia and other non-nutritive sweeteners such as Swerve
- Ketchup (Sugar-free)
- Dark chocolate/cocoa

FOODS TO AVOID

Bread and Grains

Bread is a staple food in many countries. You have loaves, bagels, tortillas, and the list goes on. However, no matter what form bread takes, they still contain a lot of carbs. The same applies to whole-grain as well because they are made from refined flour.

Depending on your daily carb limit, eating a sandwich or bagel can put your way over your daily limit. So if you want to eat bread, it is best to make keto variants at home instead. Grains such as rice, wheat, and oats contain a lot of carbs too.

So limit or avoid that as well.

Some Fruits

Fruits are healthy for you. They are found to make you have a lower risk of heart disease and cancer. However, there are a few that you need to avoid in your keto diet.

The problem is that some of those foods contain quite a lot of carbs, such as banana, raisins, dates, mango, and pear. As a general rule, avoid sweet and dried fruits. Berries are an exception because they do not contain as much sugar and are rich in fiber. So you can still eat some of them, around 50 g. Moderation is key.

Vegetables

You need to avoid or limit vegetables high in starch because they have more carbs than fiber. That includes corn, potato, sweet potato, and beets.

Pasta

Pasta is also a staple food in many countries. It is versatile and convenient. As with any other suitable food, pasta is rich in carbs. So when you are on your keto diet, spaghetti or many different pasta types are not recommended. You can probably eat a small portion, but that is not suggested. Thankfully, that does not mean you need to give up on it altogether. If you are craving pasta, you can try some other low-in carbs such as spiralized veggies or shirataki noodles.

Cereal

Cereal is also a massive offender because sugary breakfast cereals contain a lot of carbs. That also applies to "healthy cereals." Just because they use other words to describe their product does not mean that you should believe them. That also applies to oatmeal, whole-grain cereals, etc. So if you get your cereal when you are doing keto, you are already way over your carb limit, and we haven't even added milk into the equation!

Therefore, avoid whole-grain cereal or cereals that we mention here altogether.

CHAPTER 5: Working Out The Gym And Weights Are Important To Firm Up The "Skinny Fat"!

Even when you are 50 and older, there are still so many exercise options that are crucial for strengthening your body and keeping you fit. Of course, you won't be bench-pressing 150 pounds, but what we will list here may already be something that you have considered doing.

Yoga

Yoga is likely one of the most recommended exercises for everyone, especially those over 50. Yoga keeps your body flexible, limber and also calms your mind.

It does sound weird because not many people would think of yoga as an ideal exercise option, but hear us out. You may think of yoga as people bending themselves into a pretzel. But the idea behind yoga is to strengthen your focus, balance, and flexibility. Even if your arms or legs stiffen up at a certain point, there are alternative moves to help you ease into the exercise.

Overall, yoga helps you maintain a fit body and a calm mind. Also, it can help regulate your blood pressure and balance your nervous system using various breathing techniques. When was the last time you breathed deeply?

Weight Training

Again, you won't be bench-pressing 150 pounds. Weight training is still a crucial exercise at any age because you always will be picking up, moving around, and putting things down. It would help if you toned down on how much you lift to compensate for your lack of muscle mass and strength,

There is no definitive starting point here. It would be best if you did some exploring to know where your limit is, so start light and work your way up to heavier weight. Aim for the value that is just light enough to allow you to do 10 reps where the final few reps become challenging. If you can do more than 10, increase the weight. If you cannot reach 10, move down the weight range.

Lifting weight will help you build your muscle to compensate for the lost mass and keep your body healthy. Twice a week try to do weight training for each muscle group to keep your strength evenly strengthened throughout your body.

Other than that, there are a few things you need to watch out for. Do not exercise the same muscle group two days in a row. Give it time to rest because it only gets stronger when it is resting after an exercise. Also, if you feel any pain, stop or try lighter weight.

Alternatively, if barbells and dumbbells seem intimidating to you, you can try out the following:

- Resistance bands
- Exercise equipment
- Pushups
- Modified squats and lunges

Swimming

Swimming is an excellent alternative to strength training because you will not be straining your joints and the rest of your body as much. Plus, you will still get the benefit of toning your muscles and increase your flexibility. Swimming is also an aerobic activity, meaning that your heart and blood flow will also benefit from this. Just like yoga, swimming also helps you relieve stress and improve your mood.

If you wish to take it a step further, give water aerobics a shot. You might enjoy it so much that it is not even an exercise for you!

Cycling

Cycling is just as easy on your joints. It helps lower the risk of heart attacks, regulate blood pressure, and help your mood. Cycling is quite useful if you have back, neck, or shoulder pains to use a stationary recumbent bicycle.

Such a device is very ergonomically comfortable because you can rest your arms and back in a comfortable position while moving your legs. Of course, to get the full benefit of cycling, you should visit bike trails. As an added benefit, you get to enjoy the beautiful natural scenery.

Pilates

If you're suffering from back pain, then you need to perform exercises that strengthen the core. In this case, Pilates will work miracles on your body.

Simply put, Pilates is all about creating long, lean muscles and conditioning your body by using controlled movements. It strengthens, lengthens, and tones all core and stabilization areas while increasing your flexibility, range of motion, and perfecting your posture. Moreover, Pilates is straightforward because there are alternative exercises to help beginners with incredibly stiff limbs.

MEASUREMENT CONVERSION

Volume Equivalents (Liquid)

Type	US Standard (ounces)	Metric
2 tablespoons	1 fl. oz.	30 mL
¼ cup	2 fl. oz.	60 mL
½ cup	4 fl. oz.	120 mL
1 cup	8 fl. oz.	240mL

Volume Equivalents (Dry)

Type	Metric
¼ teaspoon	1 mL
½ teaspoon	2 mL
1 teaspoon	5 mL
1 tablespoon	15 mL
¼ cup	59 mL
½ cup	118 mL
1 cup	235 mL

Oven Temperatures

Fahrenheit (°F)	Celsius (°C)
250	120
300	150
325	165
350	180
375	190
400	200
425	220
450	230

BREAKFAST RECIPES

CHEESE CREPES

Prep.: 15 min. | **Cook:** 20 min. | **Servings:** 5

Ingredients:

- 6 ounces cream cheese, softened
- 1/3 cup Parmesan cheese, grated
- 6 large organic eggs
- 1 teaspoon granulated Erythritol
- 1½ tablespoon coconut flour
- 1/8 teaspoon xanthan gum
- 2 tablespoons unsalted butter

Directions:

1. In a blender, add cream cheese, Parmesan cheese, eggs, and erythritol and pulse on low speed until well combined.
2. While the motor is running, place the coconut flour and xanthan gum and pulse until a thick mixture is formed.
3. Now, pulse on medium speed for a few seconds.
4. Transfer the mixture into a bowl then set aside for about 5 minutes.
5. Divide the mixture into 10 equal-sized portions.
6. In a nonstick pan, melt butter over medium-low heat.
7. Place 1 portion of the mixture and tilt the pan to spread into a thin layer.
8. Cook for about 1½ minutes or until the edges become brown.
9. Flip the crepe and cook for about 15-20 seconds more.
10. Repeat with the remaining mixture.
11. Serve warm with your favorite keto-friendly filling.

Nutritional Information per Serving:

Cal. 297 cal - Fats 25.1 g - Carbs 3.5 g - Prot. 13.7 g

RICOTTA PANCAKES

Prep.: 10 min. | **Cook:** 20 min. | **Servings:** 4

Ingredients:

- 4 organic eggs
- ½ cup ricotta cheese
- ¼ cup unsweetened vanilla whey protein powder
- ½ teaspoon organic baking powder
- Pinch of salt
- ½ teaspoon liquid stevia
- 2 tablespoons unsalted butter

Directions:

1. Using a blender, add all the ingredients and pulse until well combined.
2. In a wok, melt butter over medium heat.
3. Add the desired amount of the mixture and spread it evenly.
4. Cook for about 2–3 minutes or until bottom becomes golden-brown.
5. Flip and cook for about 1–2 minutes or until golden brown.
6. Repeat with the remaining mixture.
7. Serve warm.

Nutritional Information per Serving:

Cal. 184 - Fats 12.9 g - Carbs 2.7 g - Prot. 14 g

Yogurt Waffles

Prep.: 15 min. | **Cook:** 25 min. | **Servings:** 5

Ingredients:

- ½ cup golden flax seeds meal
- ½ cup plus 3 tablespoons almond flour
- 1-1½ tablespoons granulated erythritol
- 1 tablespoon unsweetened vanilla whey protein powder
- ¼ teaspoon baking soda
- ½ teaspoon organic baking powder
- ¼ teaspoon xanthan gum
- Salt, as required
- 1 large organic egg, white and yolk separated
- 1 organic whole egg
- 2 tablespoons unsweetened almond milk
- 1½ tablespoons unsalted butter
- 3 ounces plain Greek yogurt

Directions:

1. Preheat the waffle iron and grease it.
2. In a large bowl, add the flour, erythritol, protein powder, baking soda, baking powder, xanthan gum, and salt, and mix until well combined.
3. Using a second small bowl, add the egg white and beat until stiff peaks form.
4. In a third bowl, add 2 egg yolks, whole egg, almond milk, butter, and yogurt, and beat until well combined.
5. Place egg mixture into the bowl of flour mixture and mix until well combined.
6. Gently, fold in the beaten egg whites.
7. Place ¼ cup of the mixture into preheated waffle iron and cook for about 4–5 minutes or until golden-brown.
8. Repeat with the remaining mixture.
9. Serve warm.

Nutritional Information per Serving:

Cal. 250 - Fats 18.7 g - Carbs 8.8 g - Prot. 8.4 g

Broccoli Muffins

Prep.: 15 min. | **Cook:** 20 min. | **Servings:** 6

Ingredients:

- 2 tablespoons unsalted butter
- 6 large organic eggs
- ½ cup heavy whipping cream
- ½ cup Parmesan cheese, grated
- Salt and ground black pepper, as required
- 1¼ cups broccoli, chopped
- 2 tablespoons fresh parsley, chopped
- ½ cup Swiss cheese, grated

Directions:

1. Preheat your oven to 350°F.
2. Grease a 12-cup muffin tin.
3. In a bowl, you will add the eggs, cream, Parmesan cheese, salt, and black pepper, and beat until well combined.
4. Divide the broccoli and parsley in the bottom of each prepared muffin cup evenly.
5. Top with the egg mixture, followed by the Swiss cheese.
6. Bake for about 20 minutes, rotating the pan once halfway through.
7. Remove from the oven and then place onto a wire rack for about 5 minutes before serving.
8. Carefully, invert the muffins onto a serving platter and serve warm.

Nutritional Information per Serving:

Cal. 231 - Fats 18 g - Carbs 2.5 g - Prot. 13.5 g

Pumpkin Bread

Prep.: 15 min. | **Cook:** 1 hour | **Servings:** 16

Ingredients:

- 1 2/3 cups almond flour
- 1½ teaspoons organic baking powder
- ½ teaspoon pumpkin pie spice
- ½ teaspoon ground cinnamon
- ½ teaspoon ground cloves
- ½ teaspoon salt
- 8 ounces cream cheese, softened
- 6 organic eggs, divided
- 1 tablespoon coconut flour
- 1 cup powdered erythritol, divided
- 1 teaspoon stevia powder, divided
- 1 teaspoon organic lemon extract
- 1 cup homemade pumpkin puree
- ½ cup coconut oil, melted

Directions:

1. Preheat your oven to 325°F.
2. Lightly, grease 2 bread loaf pans.
3. In a bowl, place almond flour, baking powder, spices, and salt, and mix until well combined.
4. In a second bowl, add the cream cheese, 1 egg, coconut flour, ¼ cup of erythritol, and ¼ teaspoon of the stevia, and with a wire whisk, beat until smooth.
5. In a third bowl, add the pumpkin puree, oil, 5 eggs, ¾ cup of the erythritol and ¾ teaspoon of the stevia and with a wire whisk, beat until well combined.
6. Add the pumpkin mixture into the bowl of the flour mixture and mix until just combined.
7. Place about ¼ of the pumpkin mixture into each loaf pan evenly.
8. Top each pan with the cream cheese mixture evenly, followed by the remaining pumpkin mixture.
9. Bake for about 50–60 minutes or until a toothpick inserted in the center comes out clean.
10. Remove the bread pans from oven and place onto a wire rack to cool for about 10 minutes.
11. Now, invert each bread loaf onto the wire rack to cool completely before slicing.
12. With a sharp knife, cut each bread loaf in the desired-sized slices and serve.

Nutritional Information per Serving:

Cal. 216 - Fats 19.8 g - Carbs 4.5 g - Prot. 3.4 g

Eggs in Avocado Cups

Prep.: 10 min. | **Cook:** 20 min. | **Servings:** 4

Ingredients:

- 2 ripe avocados, halved and pitted
- 4 organic eggs
- Salt and ground black pepper, as required
- 4 tablespoons cheddar cheese, shredded
- 2 cooked bacon slices, chopped
- 1 tablespoon scallion greens, chopped

Directions:

1. Preheat your oven to 400°F.
2. Carefully, remove abut about 2 tablespoons of flesh from each avocado half.
3. Place avocado halves into a small baking dish.
4. Carefully, crack an egg in each avocado half and sprinkle with salt and black pepper.
5. Top each egg with cheddar cheese evenly.
6. Bake for about 20 minutes or until desired doneness of the eggs.
7. Serve immediately with the garnishing of bacon and chives.

Nutritional Information per Serving:

Cal. 343 - Fats 29 g - Carbs 7.9 g - Prot. 13.8 g

CHEDDAR SCRAMBLE

Prep.: 10 min. | **Cook:** 8 min. | **Servings:** 6

Ingredients:

- 2 tablespoons olive oil
- 1 small yellow onion, chopped finely
- 12 large organic eggs, beaten lightly
- Salt and ground black pepper, as required
- 4 ounces cheddar cheese, shredded

Directions:

1. In a large wok, heat oil over medium heat and sauté the onion for about 4–5 minutes.
2. Add the eggs, salt, and black pepper and cook for about 3 minutes, stirring continuously.
3. Remove from the heat and immediately, stir in the cheese.
4. Serve immediately.

Nutritional Information per Serving:

Cal. 264 - Fats 20 g - Carbs 2.1 g - Prot. 17 g

BACON OMELET

Prep.: 10 min. | **Cook:** 15 min. | **Servings:** 2

Ingredients:

- 4 large organic eggs
- 1 tablespoon fresh chives, minced
- Salt and ground black pepper, as required
- 4 bacon slices
- 1 tablespoon unsalted butter
- 2 ounces cheddar cheese, shredded

Directions:

1. In a bowl, add the eggs, chives, salt, and black pepper, and beat until well combined.

2. Heat a non-stick frying pan over medium-high heat and cook the bacon slices for about 8–10 minutes.
3. To drain place, the bacon onto a paper towel-lined plate. Then chop the bacon slices.
4. With paper towels, wipe out the frying pan.
5. In the same frying pan, melt butter over medium-low heat and cook the egg mixture for about 2 minutes.
6. Carefully, flip the omelet and top with chopped bacon.
7. Cook for 1–2 minutes or until desired doneness of eggs.
8. Remove from heat and immediately, place the cheese in the center of omelet.
9. Fold the edges of omelet over cheese and cut into 2 portions.
10. Serve immediately.

Nutritional Information per Serving:

Cal. 427 - Fats 28.2 g - Carbs 1.2 g - Prot. 29 g

SHEET PAN EGGS WITH VEGGIES AND PARMESAN

Prep.: 5 min. | **Cook:** 15 min. | **Servings:** 6

Ingredients:

- 12 large eggs, whisked
- Salt and pepper
- 1 small red pepper, diced
- 1 small yellow onion, chopped
- 1 cup diced mushrooms
- 1 cup diced zucchini
- 1 cup freshly grated parmesan cheese

Directions:

1. Preheat the oven to 350°F and grease a rimmed baking sheet with cooking spray.
2. Whisk the eggs in a bowl with salt and pepper until frothy.

3. Stir in the peppers, onions, mushrooms, and zucchini until well combined.
4. Pour the mixture in the baking sheet and spread into an even layer.
5. Sprinkle with parmesan and bake for 12 to 15 minutes until the egg is set.
6. Let cool slightly, then cut into squares to serve.

Nutritional Information per Serving:

Cal. 215 - Fats 14 g - Carbs 5 g - Prot. 18.5 g

ALMOND BUTTER MUFFINS

Prep.: 10 min. | **Cook:** 25 min. | **Servings:** 12

Ingredients:

- 2 cups almond flour
- 1 cup powdered erythritol
- 2 teaspoons baking powder
- ¼ teaspoon salt
- ¾ cup almond butter, warmed
- ¾ cup unsweetened almond milk
- 4 large eggs

Directions:

1. Preheat the oven to 350°F and line a muffin pan with paper liners.
2. Whisk the almond flour together with the erythritol, baking powder, and salt in a mixing bowl.
3. In a separate bowl, whisk together the almond milk, almond butter, and eggs.
4. Stir the wet ingredients into the dry until just combined.
5. Spoon the batter into the prepared pan and bake for 22 to 25 minutes until a knife inserted in the center comes out clean.
6. Cool the muffins in the pan for 5 minutes then turn out onto a wire cooling rack.

Nutritional Information per Serving:

Cal. 135 - Fats 11 g - Carbs 4 g - Prot. 6 g

CLASSIC WESTERN OMELET

Prep.: 5 min. | **Cook:** 10 min. | **Servings:** 1

Ingredients:

- 2 teaspoons coconut oil
- 3 large eggs, whisked
- 1 tablespoon heavy cream
- Salt and pepper
- ¼ cup diced green pepper
- ¼ cup diced yellow onion
- ¼ cup diced ham

Directions:

1. Whisk together the eggs, heavy cream, salt and pepper in a small bowl.
2. Heat 1 teaspoon coconut oil in a small skillet over medium heat.
3. Add the peppers, onions, and ham then sauté for 3 to 4 minutes.
4. Spoon the mixture into a bowl and reheat the skillet with the rest of the oil.
5. Pour in the whisked eggs and cook until the bottom of the egg starts to set.
6. Tilt the pan to spread the egg and cook until almost set.
7. Spoon the veggie and ham mixture over half the omelet and fold it over.
8. Let the omelet cook until the eggs are set then serve hot.

Nutritional Information per Serving:

Cal. 415 - Fats 32.5 g - Carbs 6.5 g - Prot. 25 g

SHEET PAN EGGS WITH HAM AND PEPPER JACK

Prep.: 5 min. | **Cook:** 15 min. | **Servings:** 6

Ingredients:

- 12 large eggs, whisked

- Salt and pepper
- 2 cups diced ham
- 1 cup shredded pepper jack cheese

Directions:

1. Preheat the oven to 350°F and grease a rimmed baking sheet with cooking spray.
2. Whisk the eggs in a bowl with salt and pepper until frothy.
3. Stir in the ham and cheese until well combined.
4. Pour the mixture in the baking sheet and spread into an even layer.
5. Bake for 12 to 15 minutes until the egg is set.
6. Let cool slightly then cut into squares to serve.

Nutritional Information per Serving:

Cal. 235 g - Fats 15 g - Carbs 2.5 g - Prot. 21 g

CRISPY CHAI WAFFLES

Prep.: 10 min. | **Cook:** 20 min. | **Servings:** 4

Ingredients:

- 4 large eggs, separated into whites and yolks
- 3 tablespoons coconut flour
- 3 tablespoons powdered erythritol
- 1 ¼ teaspoon baking powder
- 1 teaspoon vanilla extract
- ½ teaspoon ground cinnamon
- ¼ teaspoon ground ginger
- Pinch ground cloves
- Pinch ground cardamom
- 3 tablespoons coconut oil, melted
- 3 tablespoons unsweetened almond milk

Directions:

1. Separate the eggs into two different mixing bowls.
2. Whip the egg whites until stiff peaks form then set aside.

3. Whisk the egg yolks with the coconut flour, erythritol, baking powder, vanilla, cinnamon, cardamom, and cloves in the other bowl.
4. Add the melted coconut oil to the second bowl while whisking then whisk in the almond milk.
5. Gently fold in the egg whites until just combined.
6. Preheat the waffle iron and grease with cooking spray.
7. Spoon about ½ cup of batter into the iron.
8. Cook the waffle according to the manufacturer's instructions.
9. Remove the waffle to a plate and repeat with the remaining batter.

Nutritional Information per Serving:

Cal. 215 - Fats 17 g - Carbs 8 g - Prot. 8 g

BACON CHEESEBURGER WAFFLES

Prep.: 10 Min. | **Cook:** 20 Min. | **Servings:** 4

Ingredients:

Toppings

- Pepper and Salt to taste
- 1.5 ounces of cheddar cheese
- 4 tablespoons of sugar-free barbecue sauce
- 4 slices of bacon
- 4 ounces of ground beef, 70% lean meat and 30% fat

Waffle dough

- Pepper and salt to taste
- 3 tablespoons of parmesan cheese, grated
- 4 tablespoons of almond flour
- ¼ teaspoon of onion powder
- ¼ teaspoon of garlic powder
- 1 cup (125 g) of cauliflower crumbles
- 2 large eggs
- 1.5 ounces of cheddar cheese

Directions:

1. Shred about 3 ounces of cheddar cheese then add in cauliflower crumbles in a bowl and put in a half of the cheddar cheese.
2. Put into the mixture spices, almond flour, eggs and parmesan cheese then mix and put aside for some time.
3. Thinly slice the bacon and cook in a skillet on medium to high heat.
4. After the bacon is cooked partially, put in the beef. Cook until the mixture is well done.
5. Then put the excess grease from the bacon mixture into the waffle mixture. Set aside the bacon mix.
6. Use an immersion blender to blend the waffle mix until it becomes a paste then add into the waffle iron half of the mix and cook until it becomes crispy.
7. Repeat for the remaining waffle mixture.
8. As the waffles cook, add sugar-free barbecue sauce to the ground beef and bacon mixture in the skillet.
9. Then proceed to assemble waffles by topping them with half of the left cheddar cheese and half the beef mixture. Repeat this for the remaining waffles, broil for around 1-2 minutes until the cheese has melted then serve right away.

Nutritional Information per Serving:

Cal. 405 - Fats 33 g - Carbs 4.5 - Prot. 18.8 g

KETO BREAKFAST CHEESECAKE

Prep.: 20 Min. | **Cook:** 45 Min. | **Servings:** 24

Ingredients:

Toppings

- 1/4 cup of mixed berries for each cheesecake, frouncesen and thawed

Filling ingredients:

- ½ teaspoon of vanilla extract
- ½ teaspoon of almond extract
- 3/4 cup of sweetener
- 6 eggs
- 8 ounces of cream cheese
- 16 ounces of cottage cheese

Crust ingredients:

- 4 tablespoons of salted butter
- 2 tablespoons of sweetener
- 2 cups of almonds, whole

Directions:

- Preheat oven to around 350°F.
- Pulse almonds in a food processor then add in butter and sweetener.
- Pulse until all the ingredients mix well.
- Coat twelve silicone muffin pans using foil or paper liners.
- Divide the batter evenly between the muffin pans then press into the bottom part until it forms a crust and bake for about 8 minutes.
- In the meantime, mix in a food processor the cream cheese and cottage cheese then pulse until the mixture is smooth.
- Put in the extracts and sweetener then combine until well mixed.
- Add in eggs and pulse again until it becomes smooth; you might need to scrape down the mixture from the sides of the processor. Share equally the batter between the muffin pans, then bake for around 30-40 minutes until the middle is not wobbly when you shake the muffin pan lightly.
- Put aside until cooled completely then put in the refrigerator for about 2 hours and then top with frouncesen and thawed berries.

Nutritional Information per Serving:

Cal. 152 - Fats 12 g - Carbs 3 g - Prot. 6 g

KETO EGG-CRUST PIZZA

Prep.: 5 Min. | **Cook:** 15 Min. | **Servings:** 1-2

Ingredients:

- ¼ teaspoon of dried oregano to taste
- ½ teaspoon of spike seasoning to taste
- 1 ounce of mozzarella, chopped into small cubes
- 6 – 8 sliced thinly black olives
- 6 slices of turkey pepperoni, sliced into half
- 4-5 thinly sliced small grape tomatoes
- 2 eggs, beaten well
- 1-2 teaspoons of olive oil

Directions:

1. Preheat the broiler in an oven then in a small bowl, beat well the eggs.
2. Cut the pepperoni and tomatoes in slices then cut the mozzarella cheese into cubes.
3. Put some olive oil in a skillet over medium heat then heat the pan for around one minute until it begins to get hot.
4. Add in eggs and season with oregano and spike seasoning then cook for around 2 minutes until the eggs begin to set at the bottom.
5. Drizzle half of the mozzarella, olives, pepperoni and tomatoes on the eggs followed by another layer of the remaining half of the above ingredients.
6. Ensure that there is a lot of cheese on the topmost layers.
7. Cover the skillet using a lid and cook until the cheese begins to melt and the eggs are set, for around 3-4 minutes.
8. Place the pan under the preheated broiler, cook until the top gets brown color and the cheese has melted nicely for around 2-3 minutes.
9. Serve immediately.

Nutritional Information per Serving:

Cal. 363 - Fats 24 g - Carbs 20 g - Prot. 19.2 g

BREAKFAST ROLL-UPS

Prep.: 5 Min. | **Cook:** 15 Min. | **Servings:** 5 roll-ups

Ingredients:

- Non-stick cooking spray
- 5 patties of cooked breakfast sausage
- 5 slices of cooked bacon
- 1.5 cups of cheddar cheese, shredded
- Pepper and salt
- 10 large eggs

Directions:

1. Preheat a skillet on medium to high heat then using a whisk, combine together two of the eggs in a mixing bowl. After the pan has become hot, lower the heat to medium-low heat then put in the eggs. If you want to, you can utilize some cooking spray. Season eggs with some pepper and salt.
2. Cover the eggs and leave them to cook for a couple of minutes.
3. Drizzle around 1/3 cup of cheese on top of the eggs then place a strip of bacon and divide the sausage into two and place on top.
4. Roll the eggs carefully on top of the fillings. The roll-up will almost look like a taquito. If you have a hard time folding over the eggs, use a spatula to keep them intact until they have molded into a roll-up.
5. Put aside the roll-up then repeat the above steps until you have four more roll-ups; you should have 5 roll-ups in total.

Nutritional Information per Serving:

Cal. 412 - Fats 31 g - Carbs 2.2 g - Prot. 28.2 g

Frozen Keto Coffee

Prep.: 5 min. | **Cook:** 20 min. | **Servings:** 1

Ingredients:

- 12 ounces coffee, chilled
- 1 scoop MCT powder (or 1 tablespoon MCT oil)
- 1 tablespoon heavy (whipping) cream
- Pinch ground cinnamon
- Dash sweetener (optional)
- ½ cup ice

Directions:

1. In a blender, combine the coffee, MCT powder, cream, cinnamon, sweetener (if using), and ice.
2. Blend until smooth.

Nutritional Information per Serving:

Cal. 127 - Fats 13 g - Carbs 1.5 g - Prot. 1 g

No-Bake Keto Power Bars

Prep.: 10 Min. | **Cook:** 0 min. | **Servings:** 12 bars

Ingredients:

- ½ cup pili nuts
- ½ cup whole hazelnuts
- ½ cup walnut halves
- ¼ cup hulled sunflower seeds
- ¼ cup unsweetened coconut flakes or chips
- ¼ cup hulled hemp seeds
- 2 tablespoons unsweetened cacao nibs
- 2 scoops collagen powder (I use 1 scoop Perfect Keto vanilla collagen and 1 scoop Perfect Keto unflavored collagen powder)
- ½ teaspoon ground cinnamon
- ½ teaspoon sea salt
- ¼ cup coconut oil, melted
- 1 teaspoon vanilla extract
- Stevia or monk fruit to sweeten (optional if you are using unflavored collagen powder)

Directions:

1. Line a 9-inch square baking pan with parchment paper.
2. In a food processor or blender, combine the pili nuts, hazelnuts, walnuts, sunflower seeds, coconut, hemp seeds, cacao nibs, collagen powder, cinnamon, and salt and pulse a few times.
3. Add the coconut oil, vanilla extract, and sweetener (if using). Pulse again until the ingredients are combined. Do not over pulse or it will turn to mush. You want the nuts and seeds to have some texture still.
4. Pour the mixture into the prepared pan and press it into an even layer. Cover with another piece of parchment (or fold over extra from the first piece) and place a heavy pot or dish on top to help press the bars together.
5. Refrigerate overnight and then cut into 12 bars. Store the bars in individual storage bags in the refrigerator for a quick grab-and-go breakfast.

Nutritional Information per Serving:

Cal. 242 - Fats 22 g - Carbs 4.5 g - Prot. 6.5 g

Easy Skillet Pancakes

Prep.: 5 min. | **Cook:** 5 min. | **Servings:** 8

Ingredients:

- 8 ounces cream cheese
- 8 eggs
- 2 tablespoons coconut flour
- 2 teaspoons baking powder
- 1 teaspoon ground cinnamon
- ½ teaspoon vanilla extract
- 1 teaspoon liquid stevia or sweetener of choice (optional)
- 2 tablespoons butter

Directions:

1. In a blender, combine the cream cheese, eggs, coconut flour, baking powder, cinnamon, vanilla, and stevia (if using). Blend until smooth.
2. In a large skillet over medium heat, melt the butter.
3. Use half the mixture to pour four evenly sized pancakes and cook for about a minute, until you see bubbles on top. Flip the pancakes and cook for another minute. Remove from the pan and add more butter or oil to the skillet if needed. Repeat with the remaining batter.
4. Top with butter and eat right away, or freeze the pancakes in a freezer-safe resealable bag with sheets of parchment in between, for up to 1 month.

Nutritional Information per Serving:

Cal. 179 - Fats 15 g - Carbs 3 g - Prot. 8 g

Quick Keto Blender Muffins

Prep.: 5 min. | **Cook:** 25 min. | **Servings:** 12

Ingredients:

- Butter, ghee, or coconut oil for greasing the pan
- 6 eggs
- 8 ounces cream cheese, at room temperature
- 2 scoops flavored collagen powder
- 1 teaspoon ground cinnamon
- 1 teaspoon baking powder
- Few drops or dash sweetener (optional)

Directions:

1. Preheat the oven to 350°F. Grease a 12-cup muffin pan very well with butter, ghee, or coconut oil.
2. Alternatively, you can use silicone cups or paper muffin liners.
3. In a blender, combine the eggs, cream cheese, collagen powder, cinnamon, baking powder, and sweetener (if using).
4. Blend until well combined and pour the mixture into the muffin cups, dividing equally.
5. Bake for 22 to 25 minutes until the muffins are golden brown on top and firm.
6. Let cool then store in a glass container or plastic bag in the refrigerator for up to 2 weeks or in the freezer for up to 3 months.
7. To servings refrigerated muffins, heat in the microwave for 30 seconds.
8. To meals from frozen, thaw in the refrigerator overnight and then microwave for 30 seconds, or microwave straight from the freezer for 45 to 60 seconds or until heated through.

Nutritional Information per Serving:

Cal. 120 - Fats 10 g - Carbs 1.5 g - Prot. 6 g

KETO EVERYTHING BAGELS

Prep.: 10 min. | **Cook:** 15 min. | **Servings:** 8

Ingredients:

- 2 cups shredded mozzarella cheese
- 2 tablespoons labneh cheese (or cream cheese)
- 1½ cups almond flour
- 1 egg
- 2 teaspoons baking powder
- ¼ teaspoon sea salt
- 1 tablespoon Everything Seasoning

Directions:

1. Preheat the oven to 400°F.
2. In a microwave-safe bowl, combine the mozzarella and labneh cheeses.
3. Microwave for 30 seconds, stir, then microwave for another 30 seconds.
4. Stir well.
5. If not melted completely, microwave for another 10 to 20 seconds.
6. Add the almond flour, egg, baking powder, and salt to the bowl and mix well. Form into a dough using a spatula or your hands.
7. Cut the dough into 8 roughly equal pieces and form into balls.
8. Roll each dough ball into a cylinder, then pinch the ends together to seal.
9. Place the dough rings in a nonstick donut pan or arrange them on a parchment paper–lined baking sheet.
10. Sprinkle with the seasoning and bake for 12 to 15 minutes or until golden brown.
11. Store in plastic bags in the freezer and defrost overnight in the refrigerator.
12. Reheat in the oven or toaster for a quick grab-and-go breakfast.

Nutritional Information per Serving:

Cal. 241 - Fats 19 g - Carbs 5.5 g - Prot. 12 g

TURMERIC CHICKEN AND KALE SALAD WITH FOOD, LEMON AND HONEY

Prep.: 20 min. | **Cook:** 15 min. | **Servings:** 4

Ingredients:

For the chicken:

- 1 teaspoon of clarified butter or 1 tablespoon of coconut oil
- ½ medium brown onion, diced
- 9 ounces minced chicken meat or diced chicken legs
- 1 large garlic clove, diced
- 1 teaspoon of turmeric powder
- 1 teaspoon of lime zest
- ½ lime juice
- ½ teaspoon of salt + pepper

For the salad:

- 6 stalks of broccoli or 2 cups of broccoli flowers
- 2 tablespoons of pumpkin seeds (seeds)
- 3 large cabbage leaves, stems removed and chopped
- ½ sliced avocado
- Handful of fresh coriander leaves, chopped
- Handful of fresh parsley leaves, chopped

For the dressing:

- 3 tablespoons of lime juice
- 1 small garlic clove, diced or grated
- 3 tablespoons of virgin olive oil (I used 1 tablespoon of avocado oil and 2 tablespoons of EVO)
- 1 teaspoon of raw honey
- ½ teaspoon whole or Dijon mustard
- ½ teaspoon of sea salt with pepper

Directions:

1. Heat the coconut oil in a pan. Add the onion and sauté over medium heat for 4-5 minutes, until golden brown. Add the minced chicken and garlic and stir 2-3 minutes over medium-high heat, separating.
2. Add your turmeric, lime zest, lime juice, salt and pepper, and cook, stirring consistently, for another 3-4 minutes.
3. Set the ground beef aside.
4. While your chicken is cooking, put a small saucepan of water to the boil. Add your broccoli and cook for 2 minutes.
5. Rinse with cold water and cut into 3-4 pieces each.
6. Add the pumpkin seeds to the chicken pan and toast over medium heat for 2 minutes, frequently stirring to avoid burning.
7. Season with a little salt.
8. Set aside. Raw pumpkin seeds are also good to use.
9. Put the chopped cabbage in a salad bowl and pour it over the dressing.
10. Using your hands, mix, and massage the cabbage with the dressing. This will soften the cabbage, a bit like citrus juice with fish or beef Carpaccio: it "cooks" it a little.
11. Finally, mix the cooked chicken, broccoli, fresh herbs, pumpkin seeds, and avocado slices.

Nutritional Information per Serving:

Cal. 232 - Fats 11 g - Carbs 8 g - Prot. 14 g

BUCKWHEAT SPAGHETTI WITH CHICKEN CABBAGE AND SAVORY FOOD RECIPES IN MASS SAUCE

Prep.: 15 min. | **Cook:** 15 min. | **Servings:** 2

Ingredients:

For the noodles:

- 2-3 handfuls of cabbage leaves (removed from the stem and cut)
- Buckwheat noodles 150g / 5oz (100% buckwheat, without wheat)
- 3-4 shiitake mushrooms, sliced
- 1 teaspoon of coconut oil or butter
- 1 brown onion, finely chopped
- 1 medium chicken breast, sliced or diced
- 1 long red pepper, thinly sliced
- 2 large garlic cloves, diced
- 2-3 tablespoons of Tamari sauce (gluten-free soy sauce)

For the miso dressing:

- 1 tablespoon and a half of fresh organic miso
- 1 tablespoon of Tamari sauce
- 1 tablespoon of extra virgin olive oil
- 1 tablespoon of lemon or lime juice
- 1 teaspoon of sesame oil (optional)

Directions:

1. Boil a medium saucepan of water.
2. Add the black cabbage and cook 1 minute, until it is wilted.
3. Remove and reserve, but reserve the water and return to boiling.
4. Add your soba noodles and cook according to the directions on the package (usually about 5 minutes).
5. Rinse with cold water and reserve.
6. In the meantime, fry the shiitake mushrooms in a little butter or coconut oil (about a teaspoon) for 2-3 minutes, until its color is lightly browned on each side.
7. Sprinkle with sea salt and reserve.
8. In that same pan, heat more coconut oil or lard over medium-high heat.
9. Fry the onion and chili for 2-3 minutes, and then add the chicken pieces.
10. Cook 5 minutes on medium heat, stirring a few times, then add the garlic, tamari sauce, and a little water.

11. Cook for another 2-3 minutes, stirring continuously until your chicken is cooked.
12. Finally, add the cabbage and soba noodles and stir the chicken to warm it.
13. Stir the miso sauce and sprinkle the noodles at the end of the cooking, in this way you will keep alive all the beneficial probiotics in the miso.

Nutritional Information per Serving:

Cal. 305 - Fats 11 g - Carbs 9 g - Prot. 12 g

ASIAN KING JUMPED JAMP

Prep.: 15 min. | **Cook:** 10 min. | **Servings:** 4

Ingredients:

- 5 oz. of raw shelled prawns, not chopped
- Two teaspoons of tamari (you can use soy sauce if you don't avoid gluten)
- Two teaspoons of extra virgin olive oil
- 2.6 oz. soba (buckwheat pasta)
- 1 garlic clove, finely chopped
- 1 bird's eye chili, finely chopped
- 1 teaspoon finely chopped fresh ginger.
- 0.7 oz. of sliced red onions
- 1.4 oz. of celery, cut and sliced
- 2.6 oz. of chopped green beans
- 1.7 oz. of chopped cabbage
- ½ cup of chicken broth
- 5 g celery or celery leaves

Directions:

1. Heat a pan over high heat, and then cook the prawns in 1 teaspoon of tamari and 1 teaspoon of oil for 2-3 minutes.
2. Transfer the prawns to a plate.
3. Clean the pan with kitchen paper as it will be reused.
4. Cook your noodles in boiling water for 5-8 minutes or as indicated on the package.
5. Drain and set aside.

6. Meanwhile, fry the garlic, chili and ginger, red onion, celery, beans, and cabbage in the remaining oil over medium-high heat for 2-3 minutes.
7. Add your broth and allow it to boil, and then simmer for a minute or two, until the vegetables are cooked but crunchy.
8. Add shrimp, noodles and celery/celery leaves to the pan, bring to a boil again, then remove from the heat and serve.

Nutritional Information per Serving:

Cal. 223 - Fats 2 g - Carbs 6 g - Prot. 34 g

SPICED BUTTER WAFFLES

Prep.: 15 min. | **Cook:** 20 min. | **Servings:** 4

Ingredients:

- ½ cup super fine almond flour
- ½ teaspoon Erythritol
- ¼ teaspoon organic baking powder
- ¼ teaspoon baking soda
- ¼ teaspoon ground cinnamon
- 1/8 teaspoon ground cloves
- 1/8 teaspoon ground nutmeg
- ¼ teaspoon salt
- 2 organic eggs (whites and yolks separated)
- 2 tablespoons butter, melted
- 1 teaspoon organic vanilla extract

Directions:

1. Add flour, Erythritol, baking powder, baking soda, spices, and salt in a mixing bowl and mix well.
2. In a second bowl, add the egg yolks, butter, and vanilla, and beat until well combined.
3. In a third small glass bowl, add the egg whites and beat until soft peaks form.
4. Add the egg yolks mixture into flour mixture and mix until well combined.
5. Gently, fold in the beaten egg whites.
6. Preheat the waffle iron and then grease it.

7. Place ¼ of the mixture into preheated waffle iron and cook for about 4–5 minutes or until golden-brown.
8. Repeat with the remaining mixture.
9. Serve warm.

Nutritional Information per Serving:

Cal. 177 - Fats 15.5 g - Carbs 3.1 g - Prot. 2.8 g

CREAMY PORRIDGE

Prep.: 10 min. | **Cook:** 10 min. | **Servings:** 4

Ingredients:

- 1½ cups filtered water
- 1/3 cup almond flour
- 2 tablespoons golden flax meal
- Pinch of sea salt
- 2 organic eggs, beaten
- 2 tablespoons heavy cream
- 2 tablespoons Erythritol
- 4 teaspoons butter

Directions:

1. In a saucepan, mix together water, almond flour, ground flax, and salt until well combined.
2. Place the saucepan over medium-high heat and bring to a boil, stirring frequently.
3. Adjust the heat to medium and cook for about 2–3 minutes, beating continuously.
4. Remove the saucepan from heat and slowly, add the beaten eggs, beating continuously.
5. Return the saucepan over medium heat and cook for about 2–3 minutes or until mixture becomes thick.
6. Remove the saucepan from heat and with a wire whisk, beat the mixture for at least 30 seconds.
7. Add heavy cream, Erythritol, and butter and beat until well combined.
8. Serve immediately.

Nutritional Information per Serving:

Cal. 169 - Fats 15 g - Carbs 3.3 g - Prot. 3.7 g

CHOCOLATE PANCAKES

Prep.: 15 min. | **Cook:** 20 min. | **Servings:** 5

Ingredients:

- 4 tablespoons coconut flour
- 2 teaspoons organic baking powder
- 2 teaspoons Erythritol
- Pinch of salt
- 4 ounces cream cheese, softened
- 3 organic eggs
- 1 tablespoon organic vanilla extract
- ¼ cup unsweetened dark chocolate chips
- 2–3 tablespoons unsweetened almond milk

Directions:

1. In a blender, place all ingredients (except for almond milk) and pulse until well combined.
2. Set it aside for about 5 minutes.
3. Again, pulse for about 10 seconds.
4. Now, add almond milk and pulse until well combined.
5. Heat a lightly greased non-stick wok over medium heat.
6. Add 1/3 cup of mixture and cook for about 2 minutes or until golden-brown.
7. Flip and cook for about 1–2 minutes.
8. Repeat with the remaining mixture.
9. Serve warm.

Nutritional Information per Serving:

Cal. 231 - Fats 17.8 g - Carbs 8.5 g - Prot. 7.5 g

CREAM CREPES

Prep.: 10 min. | **Cook:** 12 min. | **Servings:** 2

Ingredients:

- 1 tablespoon butter, melted

- 2 organic eggs
- 1 teaspoon Erythritol
- 1/8 teaspoon sea salt
- 2 tablespoons coconut flour
- 1/3 cup heavy cream

Directions:

1. In a mixing bowl, add butter, eggs, Erythritol, and salt, and beat until well combined.
2. Slowly, add the flour, beating continuously until well combined.
3. Add the heavy cream and mix until blended completely.
4. Heat a lightly greased non-stick wok over medium heat.
5. Add ¼ of the mixture and tilt the pan to spread into a thin layer.
6. Cook for about 3 minutes, flipping once after 2 minutes.
7. Repeat with the remaining mixture.
8. Serve warm.

Nutritional Information per Serving:

Cal. 213 - Fats 18.5 g - Carbs 4.9 g - Prot. 7 g

ZUCCHINI MUFFINS

Prep.: 15 min. | **Cook:** 15 min. | **Servings:** 4

Ingredients:

- 4 organic eggs
- ¼ cup unsalted butter, melted
- ¼ cup water
- 1/3 cup coconut flour
- ½ teaspoon organic baking powder
- ¼ teaspoon salt
- 1½ cups zucchini, grated
- ½ cup Parmesan cheese, shredded
- 1 tablespoon fresh oregano, minced
- 1 tablespoon fresh thyme, minced
- ¼ cup cheddar cheese, grated

Directions:

1. Preheat the oven to 400°F.

2. Lightly, grease 8 muffin tins.
3. Add eggs, butter, and water in a mixing bowl and beat until well combined.
4. Add the flour, baking powder, and salt, and mix well.
5. Add remaining ingredients except for cheddar and mix until just combined.
6. Place the mixture into prepared muffin cups evenly.
7. Bake for approximately 13–15 minutes or until top of muffins become golden-brown.
8. Remove the muffin tin from oven and place onto a wire rack to cool for about 10 minutes.
9. Carefully invert the muffins onto a platter and serve warm.

Nutritional Information per Serving:

Cal. 287 - Fats 22.5 g - Carbs 9 g - Prot. 13.2 g

LEMON POPPY SEED MUFFINS

Prep.: 15 min. | **Cook:** 20 min. | **Servings:** 6

Ingredients:

- ¾ cup blanched almond flour
- ¼ cup golden flax meal
- 1/3 cup Erythritol
- 2 tablespoons poppy seeds
- 1 teaspoon organic baking powder
- 3 large organic eggs
- ¼ cup heavy cream
- ¼ cup salted butter, melted
- 3 tablespoons fresh lemon juice
- 1 teaspoon organic vanilla extract
- 20–25 drops liquid stevia
- 2 teaspoons fresh lemon zest, grated finely

Directions:

1. Preheat the oven to 350°F. Line 12 cups of a muffin tin with paper liners.
2. Add flour, flax meal, poppy seeds, Erythritol, and baking powder in a mixing bowl and mix well.

3. In another mixing bowl, add eggs, heavy cream, and butter, and beat until well combined.
4. Add egg mixture into flour mixture and mix until well combined and smooth.
5. Add lemon juice, organic vanilla extract, and liquid stevia, and mix until well combined.
6. Gently, fold in lemon zest.
7. Place the mixture into prepared muffin cups evenly.
8. Bake for approximately 18–20 minutes or until a wooden skewer inserted in the center comes out clean.
9. Remove muffin tin from oven and place onto a wire rack to cool for about 10 minutes.
10. Carefully invert the muffins onto a wire rack to cool completely before serving.

Nutritional Information per Serving:

Cal. 255 - Fats 22.6 g - Carbs 6 g - Prot. 4.9 g

BLUEBERRY BREAD

Prep.: 15 min. | **Cook:** 45 min. | **Servings:** 8

Ingredients:

- 8 large organic eggs, room temperature
- ¾ cup coconut flour
- 1/3 cup butter, melted
- 1 teaspoon organic baking powder
- 1 teaspoon organic vanilla extract
- ¼ teaspoon salt
- 1/3 cup fresh blueberries

Directions:

1. Preheat the oven to 350°F.
2. Line a 9x5-inch loaf pan with parchment paper.
3. In a food processor, add eggs and pulse on high speed until frothy.
4. Add the remaining ingredients except raspberries and pulse on high speed until smooth.

5. Transfer the mixture into a bowl and gently, fold in blueberries.
6. Place the mixture into the prepared loaf pan evenly.
7. Bake for approximately 40–45 minutes or until a wooden skewer inserted in the center comes out clean.
8. Remove the bread pan from oven and place onto a wire rack to cool for about 10 minutes.
9. Carefully, invert the bread onto the wire rack to cool completely before slicing.
10. With a sharp knife, cut the bread loaf into the desired-sized slices and serve.

Nutritional Information per Serving:

Cal. 190 - Fats 14.2 g - Carbs 7.6 g - Prot. 7.9 g

SPINACH OMELET

Prep.: 10 min. | **Cook:** 6½ min. | **Servings:** 2

Ingredients:

- 4 large organic eggs
- ¼ cup cooked spinach, squeezed
- 2 scallions, chopped
- 2 tablespoons fresh parsley, chopped
- ½ cup feta cheese, crumbled
- Ground black pepper, to taste
- 2 teaspoons butter

Directions:

1. Preheat the broiler of oven.
2. Arrange a rack about 4-inch from heating element.
3. Crack the eggs in a mixing bowl and beat well.
4. Add remaining ingredients except oil and stir to combine.
5. In an ovenproof wok, melt butter over medium heat.
6. Add egg mixture and tilt the wok to spread the mixture evenly.
7. Immediately, adjust the heat to medium-low and cook for about 3–4 minutes or until golden-brown.

8. Now, transfer the wok under broiler and broil for about 1½–2½ minutes.
9. Cut the omelet into desired size wedges and serve.

Nutritional Information per Serving:

Cal. 283 - Fats 21 g - Carbs 3.8 g - Prot. 18 g

CHEESY BREAKFAST MUFFINS

Prep.: 15 min. | **Cook:** 12 min. | **Servings:** 6

Ingredients:

- 4 tablespoons melted butter
- 3/4 tablespoon baking powder
- 1 cup almond flour
- 2 large eggs, lightly beaten
- 2 ounces cream cheese mixed with 2 tablespoons heavy whipping cream
- A handful of shredded Mexican blend cheese

Directions:

1. Preheat the oven to 400°F.
2. Grease 6 muffin tin cups with melted butter and set aside.
3. Combine the baking powder and almond flour in a bowl.
4. Stir well and set aside.
5. Stir together four tablespoons melted butter, eggs, shredded cheese, and cream cheese in a separate bowl.
6. The egg and the dry mixture must be combined using a hand mixer to beat until it is creamy and well blended.
7. The mixture must be scooped into the greased muffin cups evenly.

Nutritional Information per Serving:

Cal. 214 - Fats 15.6 g - Carbs 5.1 g - Prot. 9.5 g

SPINACH, MUSHROOM, AND GOAT CHEESE FRITTATA

Prep.: 15 min. | **Cook:** 20 min. | **Servings:** 5

Ingredients:

- 2 tablespoons olive oil
- 1 cup fresh mushrooms, sliced
- 6 bacon slices, cooked and chopped
- 1 cup spinach, shredded
- 10 large eggs, beaten
- 1/2 cup goat cheese, crumbled
- Pepper and salt

Directions:

1. Preheat the oven to 350°F.
2. Heat oil and add the mushrooms and fry for 3 minutes until they start to brown, stirring frequently.
3. Fold in the bacon and spinach and cook for about 1 to 2 minutes, or until the spinach is wilted.
4. Slowly pour in the beaten eggs and cook for 3 to 4 minutes. Making use of a spatula, lift the edges for allowing uncooked egg to flow underneath.
5. Top with the goat cheese, then sprinkle the salt and pepper to season.
6. Bake in the preheated oven for about 15 minutes until lightly golden brown around the edges.

Nutritional Information per Serving:

Cal. 265 - Fats 11 g - Carbs 5.1 g - Prot. 12 g

GREEN VEGETABLE QUICHE

Prep.: 20 min. | **Cook:** 20 min. | **Servings:** 4

Ingredients:

- 6 organic eggs
- 1/2 cup unsweetened almond milk
- Salt and ground black pepper, as required
- 2 cups fresh baby spinach, chopped
- 1/2 cup green bell pepper, seeded and chopped
- 1 scallion, chopped
- 1/4 cup fresh cilantro, chopped
- 1 tablespoon fresh chives, minced

- 3 tablespoons mozzarella cheese, grated

Directions:

1. Preheat your oven to 400°F.
2. Lightly grease a pie dish.
3. In a bowl, add eggs, almond milk, salt, and black pepper, and beat until well combined. Set aside.
4. In another bowl, add the vegetables and herbs and mix well.
5. At the bottom of the prepared pie dish, place the veggie mixture evenly and top with the egg mixture.
6. Let the quiche bake for about 20 minutes.
7. Remove the pie dish from the oven and immediately sprinkle with the Parmesan cheese.
8. Set aside for about 5 minutes before slicing.
9. Cut into desired sized wedges and serve warm.

Nutritional Information per Serving:

Cal. 298 - Fats 10.4 g - Carbs 4.1 g - Prot. 7.9 g

CHEESY BROCCOLI MUFFINS

Prep.: 15 min. | **Cook:** 20 min. | **Servings:** 6

Ingredients:

- 2 tablespoons unsalted butter
- 6 large organic eggs
- 1/2 cup heavy whipping cream
- 1/2 cup Parmesan cheese, grated
- Salt and ground black pepper, as required
- 11/4 cups broccoli, chopped
- 2 tablespoons fresh parsley, chopped
- 1/2 cup Swiss cheese, grated

Directions:

1. Grease a 12-cup muffin tin.
2. In a bowl or container, put in the cream, eggs, Parmesan cheese, salt, and black pepper, and beat until well combined.

3. Divide the broccoli and parsley in the bottom of each prepared muffin cup evenly.
4. Top with the egg mixture, followed by the Swiss cheese.
5. Let the muffins bake for about 20 minutes, rotating the pan once halfway through.
6. Carefully, invert the muffins onto a serving platter and serve warm.

Nutritional Information per Serving:

Cal. 241 - Fats 11.5 g - Carbs 4 g - Prot. 11 g

BERRY CHOCOLATE BREAKFAST BOWL

Prep.: 10 min. | **Cook:** 0 min. | **Servings:** 2

Ingredients:

- 1/2 cup strawberries, fresh or frozen
- 1/2 cup blueberries, fresh or frozen
- 1 cup unsweetened almond milk
- Sugar-free maple syrup to taste
- 2 tbsp. unsweetened cocoa powder
- 1 tbsp. cashew nuts for topping

Directions:

1. The berries must be divided into four bowls, pour on the almond milk.
2. Drizzle with the maple syrup and sprinkle the cocoa powder on top, a tablespoon per bowl.
3. Top with the cashew nuts and enjoy immediately.

Nutritional Information per Serving:

Cal. 287 - Fats 5.9 g - Carbs 3.1 g - Prot. 4.2 g

GOAT CHEESE FRITTATA

Prep.: 15 min. | **Cook:** 15 min. | **Servings:** 4

Ingredients:

- 1 tbsp. avocado oil for frying

- 2 oz. bacon slices, chopped
- 1 red bell pepper
- 1 small yellow onion, chopped
- 2 scallions, chopped
- 1 tbsp. chopped fresh chives
- Salt and black pepper to taste
- 8 eggs, beaten
- 1 tbsp. unsweetened almond milk
- 1 tbsp. chopped fresh parsley
- 3 1/2 oz. goat cheese, divided
- 3/4 oz. grated Parmesan cheese

Directions:

1. Let the oven preheat to 350°F.
2. Heat the avocado oil in a medium cast-iron pan and cook the bacon for 5 minutes or golden brown.
3. Stir in the bell pepper, onion, scallions, and chives.
4. Cook for 3 to 4 minutes or until the vegetables soften.
5. Season with salt and black pepper.
6. In a bowl or container, the eggs must be beaten with the almond milk and parsley.
7. Pour the mixture over the vegetables, stirring to spread out nicely.
8. Share half of the goat cheese on top.
9. Once the eggs start to set, divide the remaining goat cheese on top, season with salt, black pepper, and place the pan in the oven—Bake for 5 to 6 minutes or until the eggs set all around.
10. Take out the pan, scatter the Parmesan cheese on top, slice, and serve warm.

Nutritional Information per Serving:

Cal. 412 - Fats 15 g - Carbs 4.9 g - Prot. 10.5 g

LUNCH RECIPES

EASY KETO SMOKED SALMON LUNCH BOWL

Prep.: 15 min. | **Cook:** 0 min. | **Servings:** 2

Ingredients:

- 12 ounces smoked salmon
- 4 tablespoon mayonnaise
- 2 ounces spinach
- 1 tablespoon olive oil
- 1 medium lime
- Pepper
- Salt

Directions:

1. Arrange the mayonnaise, salmon, spinach on a plate.
2. Sprinkle olive oil over the spinach.
3. Serve with lime wedges and put salt plus pepper.

Nutritional Information per Serving:

Cal. 457 - Fats 34 g - Carbs 1.9 g - Prot. 32 g

EASY ONE-PAN GROUND BEEF AND GREEN BEANS

Prep.: 15 min. | **Cook:** 15 min. | **Servings:** 2

Ingredients:

- 10 ounces ground beef
- 9 ounces green beans
- Pepper
- Salt
- 2 tablespoons sour cream

- 3½ ounces butter

Directions:

1. Warm-up the butter to a pan over high heat.
2. Put the ground beef plus the pepper and salt. Cook.
3. Reduce heat to medium.
4. Add the remaining butter and the green beans then cook within five minutes.
5. Put pepper and salt, then transfer.
6. Serve with a dollop of sour cream.

Nutritional Information per Serving:

Cal. 787 - Fats 71 g - Carbs 66 g - Prot. 27 g

EASY SPINACH AND BACON SALAD

Prep.: 15 min. | **Cook:** 15 min. | **Servings:** 4

Ingredients:

- 8 ounces spinach
- 4 large hard-boiled eggs
- 6 ounces bacon
- 2 medium red onions
- 2 cups of mayonnaise
- Pepper
- Salt

Directions:

1. Cook the bacon, then chop into pieces, set aside.
2. Slice the hard-boiled eggs, and then rinse the spinach.
3. Combine the lettuce, mayonnaise, and bacon fat into a large cup, put pepper and salt.

4. Add the red onion, sliced eggs, and bacon into the salad, then toss.
5. Serve.

Nutritional Information per Serving:

Cal. 509 - Fats 46 g - Carbs 2.5 g - Prot. 19 g

EASY KETO ITALIAN PLATE

Prep.: 15 min. | **Cook:** 0 min. | **Servings:** 2

Ingredients:

- 7 ounces mozzarella cheese
- 7 ounces prosciutto
- 2 tomatoes
- 4 tablespoons olive oil
- 10 whole green olives
- Pepper
- Salt

Directions:

1. Arrange the tomato, olives, mozzarella, and prosciutto on a plate.
2. Season the tomato and cheese with pepper and salt.
3. Serve with olive oil.

Nutritional Information per Serving:

Cal. 780 - Fats 60.7 g - Carbs 6 g - Prot. 51 g

FRESH BROCCOLI AND DILL KETO SALAD

Prep.: 15 min. | **Cook:** 7 min. | **Servings:** 3

Ingredients:

- 16 ounces broccoli
- 1/2 cup mayonnaise
- 3/4 cup chopped dill
- Salt
- Pepper

Directions:

1. Boil salted water in a saucepan.
2. Put the chopped broccoli in the pot and boil for 3-5 minutes.
3. Drain and set aside.
4. Once cooled, mix the rest of the fixing.
5. Put pepper and salt, then serve.

Nutritional Information per Serving:

Cal. 303 - Fats 28.1 g - Carbs 6.2 g - Prot. 4 g

KETO SMOKED SALMON FILLED AVOCADOS

Prep.: 15 min. | **Cook:** 0 min. | **Servings:** 1

Ingredients:

- 1 avocado
- 3 ounces smoked salmon
- 4 tablespoons sour cream
- 1 tablespoon lemon juice
- Pepper
- Salt

Directions:

1. Cut the avocado into two.
2. Place the sour cream in the hollow parts of the avocado with smoked salmon.
3. Put pepper and salt, squeeze lemon juice over the top.
4. Serve.

Nutritional Information per Serving:

Cal. 517 - Fats 42 g - Carbs 6.7 g - Prot. 20 g

LOW-CARB BROCCOLI LEMON PARMESAN SOUP

Prep.: 15 min. | **Cook:** 15 min. | **Servings:** 4

Ingredients:

- 3 cups of water
- 1 cup unsweetened almond milk

- 32 ounces broccoli florets
- 1 cup heavy whipping cream
- 3/4 cup Parmesan cheese
- Salt
- Pepper
- 2 tablespoons lemon juice

Directions:

1. Cook broccoli plus water over medium-high heat.
2. Take out 1 cup of the cooking liquid, and remove the rest.
3. Blend half the broccoli, reserved cooking oil, unsweetened almond milk, heavy cream, and salt plus pepper in a blender.
4. Put the blended items to the remaining broccoli, and stir with Parmesan cheese and lemon juice.
5. Cook until heated through. Serve with Parmesan cheese on the top.

Nutritional Information per Serving:

Cal. 371 - Fats 28 g - Carbs 11 g - Prot. 14 g

PROSCIUTTO AND MOZZARELLA BOMB

Prep.: 15 min. | **Cook:** 10 min. | **Servings:** 4

Ingredients:

- 4 ounces sliced prosciutto
- 8 ounces mozzarella ball
- Olive oil

Directions:

1. Layer half of the prosciutto vertically.
2. Lay the remaining slices horizontally across the first set of slices.
3. Place mozzarella ball, upside down, onto the crisscrossed prosciutto slices.
4. Wrap the mozzarella ball with the prosciutto slices.

5. Warm-up the olive oil in a skillet, crisp the prosciutto, then serve.

Nutritional Information per Serving:

Cal. 253 - Fats 19.3 g - Carbs 1.1 g - Prot. 18 g

SUMMER TUNA AVOCADO SALAD

Prep.: 15 min. | **Cook:** 0 min. | **Servings:** 2

Ingredients:

- 1 can tuna flake
- 1 medium avocado
- 1 medium English cucumber
- ¼ cup cilantro
- 1 tbsp. lemon juice
- 1 tbsp. olive oil
- Pepper
- Salt

Directions:

1. Put the first 4 ingredients into a salad bowl.
2. Sprinkle with the lemon and olive oil.
3. Serve.

Nutritional Information per Serving:

Cal. 303 - Fats 22.6 g - Carbs 5 g - Prot. 16 g

MUSHROOMS & GOAT CHEESE SALAD

Prep.: 15 min. | **Cook:** 10 min. | **Servings:** 1

Ingredients:

- 1 tablespoon butter
- 2 ounces cremini mushrooms
- Pepper
- Salt
- 4 ounces spring mix
- 1-ounce cooked bacon
- 1-ounce goat cheese
- 1 tablespoon olive oil

- 1 tablespoon balsamic vinegar

Directions:

1. Sautee the mushrooms, put pepper and salt.
2. Place the salad greens in a bowl.
3. Top with goat cheese and crumbled bacon.
4. Mix these in the salad once the mushrooms are done.
5. Whisk the olive oil in a small bowl and balsamic vinegar.
6. Put the salad on top and serve.

Nutritional Information per Serving:

Cal. 243 - Fats 21 g - Carbs 8 g - Fiber 1 g

KETO BACON SUSHI

Prep.: 15 min. | **Cook:** 13 min. | **Servings:** 4

Ingredients:

- 6 slices bacon
- 1 avocado
- 2 Persian cucumbers
- 2 medium carrots
- 4 oz. cream cheese

Directions:

1. Warm-up oven to 400F. Line a baking sheet.
2. Place bacon halves in an even layer and bake, 11 to 13 minutes.
3. Meanwhile, slice cucumbers, avocado, and carrots into parts roughly the width of the bacon.
4. Spread an even layer of cream cheese in the cooled down bacon.
5. Divide vegetables evenly and place it on one end.
6. Roll up vegetables tightly.
7. Garnish and serve.

Nutritional Information per Serving:

Cal. 343 - Fats 30 g - Carbs 11.6 g - Prot. 28 g

COLE SLAW KETO WRAP

Prep.: 15 min. | **Cook:** 0 min. | **Servings:** 2

Ingredients:

- .3 c Red Cabbage
- .5 c Green Onions
- .75 c Mayo
- 2 tsp Apple Cider Vinegar
- 25 tsp Salt
- 16 pcs Collard Green
- 1-pound Ground Meat, cooked
- .33 c Alfalfa Sprouts
- Toothpicks

Directions:

1. Mix slaw items with a spoon in a large-sized bowl.
2. Place a collard green on a plate and scoop a tablespoon of coleslaw on the edge of the leaf.
3. Top it with a scoop of meat and sprouts.
4. Roll and tuck the sides.
5. Insert the toothpicks.
6. Serve.

Nutritional Information per Serving:

Cal. 409 - Fats 42 g - Carbs 4 g - Prot. 2 g

KETO CHICKEN CLUB LETTUCE WRAP

Prep.: 15 min. | **Cook:** 15 min. | **Servings:** 1

Ingredients:

- 1 head iceberg lettuce
- 1 tbsp. mayonnaise
- 6 slices of organic chicken
- Bacon
- Tomato

Directions:

1. Layer 6-8 large leaves of lettuce in the center of the parchment paper, around 9-10 inches.
2. Spread the mayo in the center and lay with chicken, bacon, and tomato.
3. Roll the wrap halfway through, then roll tuck in the ends of the wrap.
4. Cut it in half.
5. Serve.

Nutritional Information per Serving:

Cal. 837 - Fats 78 g - Carbs 4 g - Prot. 28 g

KETO BROCCOLI SALAD

Prep.: 10 min. | **Cook:** 0 min. | **Servings:** 4-6

Ingredients:

For salad:

- 2 broccoli
- 2 red cabbage
- .5 c sliced almonds
- 1 green onions
- .5 c raisins

For the orange almond dressing

- .33 c orange juice
- .25 c almond butter
- 2 tbsp. coconut aminos
- 1 shallot
- Salt

Directions:

1. Pulse the salt, shallot, amino, nut butter, and orange juice using a blender.
2. Combine other fixing in a bowl.
3. Toss it with dressing and serve.

Nutritional Information per Serving:

Cal. 202 - Fats 9.4 g - Carbs 1.3 g - Prot. 2.2 g

KETO SHEET PAN CHICKEN AND RAINBOW VEGGIES

Prep.: 15 min. | **Cook:** 25 min. | **Servings:** 4

Ingredients:

- Nonstick spray
- 1-pound Chicken Breasts
- 1 tbsp. Sesame Oil
- 2 tbsp. Soy Sauce
- 2 tbsp. Honey
- 2 Red Pepper
- 2 Yellow Pepper
- 3 Carrots
- ½ Broccoli
- 2 Red Onions
- 2 tbsp. EVOO
- Pepper & salt
- .25 c Parsley

Directions:

1. Grease the baking sheet, warm-up the oven to a temperature of 400°F.
2. Put the chicken in the middle of the sheet.
3. Separately, combine the oil and the soy sauce.
4. Brush over the chicken.
5. Separate veggies across the plate.
6. Sprinkle with oil and then toss.
7. Put pepper & salt.
8. Set tray into the oven and cook within 25 minutes.
9. Garnish using parsley.
10. Serve.

Nutritional Information per Serving:

Cal. 437 - Fats 30 g - Carbs 9 g - Prot. 30 g

SHRIMP LETTUCE WRAPS WITH BUFFALO SAUCE

Prep.: 15 min. | **Cook:** 20 min. | **Servings:** 4

Ingredients:

- 1 egg, beaten
- 3 Tbsp. butter
- 16 oz. shrimp, peeled, deveined, with tails removed
- ¾ cup almond flour
- ¼ cup hot sauce (like Frank's)
- 1 tsp extra-virgin olive oil
- Kosher salt
- Black pepper
- Garlic
- 1 head romaine lettuce, leaves parted, for serving
- ½ red onion, chopped
- celery, finely sliced
- ½ blue cheese, cut into pieces

Directions:

1. To make the Buffalo sauce, melt the butter in a saucepan, add the garlic and cook this mixture for 1 minute. Pour hot sauce into the saucepan and whisk to combine. Set aside.
2. In one bowl, crack one egg, add salt and pepper and mix. In another bowl, put the almond flour, add salt and pepper and also combine. Dip each shrimp into the egg mixture first and then into the almond one.
3. Take a large frying pan. Heat the oil and cook your shrimp for about 2 minutes per side.
4. Add Buffalo sauce.
5. Serve in lettuce leaves. Top your shrimp with red onion, blue cheese, and celery.

Nutritional Information per Serving:

Cal. 606 - Fats 54 g - Carbs 8 g - Prot. 33 g

POKE BOWL WITH SALMON AND VEGGIES

Prep.: 20 min. | **Cook:** 0 min. | **Servings:** 2

Ingredients:

- 8 oz. raw salmon, skinless and deboned
- 1 Tbsp. sesame oil
- 1 tsp tamari sauce
- 1 pinch salt
- 1 cup white cabbage, shredded
- 1 cup red cabbage, shredded
- ¼ cup cucumber, sliced
- 1 radish, sliced
- ½ avocado, diced
- ¼ cup cilantro
- 1 tsp white sesame seeds
- 1 tsp black sesame seeds

Directions:

1. To make the marinade, mix the sesame oil, tamari sauce and salt. Set aside.
2. Cut your salmon into cubes and put into a bowl.
3. Pour the marinade over it.
4. Place the cucumber, red and white cabbage, radish, avocado and cilantro into a bowl.
5. Add the marinated salmon.
6. Top the salmon with white and black sesame seeds.

Nutritional Information per Serving:

Cal. 446 - Fats 34 g - Carbs 11 g - Prot. 26 g

THAI CUCUMBER NOODLE SALAD

Prep.: 10 min. | **Cook:** 1 minute | **Servings:** 3

Ingredients:

- 1 cucumber, cut into noodles
- salt, to taste
- 3 pinches scallions, chopped
- 3 pinches raisins
- 3 tsp sesame seeds
- ¼ cup unsalted almond butter
- 1 tsp red curry paste
- ¼cup canned coconut milk
- 1½ Tbsp. apple cider vinegar

- ⅛ tsp coarse salt
- 1 Tbsp. coconut water

Directions:

1. With a Julienne peeler, make noodles from the cucumber.
2. To make the Thai peanut sauce, combine and mix thoroughly the unsalted almond butter, red curry paste, canned coconut milk, apple cider vinegar, coconut water, and add coarse salt.
3. Place your cucumber noodles over a spacious flat plate, pour ½ Tbsp.
4. Thai peanut sauce over the noodles.
5. Top the cucumber noodles with chopped scallions, raisins, and sesame seeds.

Nutritional Information per Serving:

Cal. 132 - Fats 10 g - Carbs 3 g - Prot. 3 g

WRAPPED BACON CHEESEBURGER

Prep.: 15 min. | **Cook:** 8 min. | **Servings:** 4

Ingredients:

- 7 oz. bacon
- 1½ pounds ground beef
- ½ tsp salt
- ¼tsp pepper
- 4 oz. cheese, shredded
- 1 head iceberg or romaine lettuce, leaves parted and washed
- 1 tomato, sliced
- ¼ pickled cucumber, finely sliced

Directions:

1. Cook bacon and set aside.
2. In a separate bowl, combine ground beef, salt, and pepper.
3. Divide mixture into 4 sections, create balls and press each one slightly to form a patty.

4. Put your patties into a frying pan and cook for about 4 minutes on each side.
5. Top each cooked patty with a slice of cheese, several pieces of bacon, and pickled cucumber.
6. Add a bit of tomato.
7. Wrap each burger in a big lettuce leaf.

Nutritional Information per Serving:

Cal. 684 - Fats 51 g - Carbs 5 g - Prot. 48 g

HEARTY LUNCH SALAD WITH BROCCOLI AND BACON

Prep.: 10 min. | **Cook:** 10 min. | **Servings:** 5

Ingredients:

- 4 cups broccoli florets, chopped
- 7 slices bacon, fried and crumbled
- ¼ cup red onion, diced
- ¼ cup almonds, sliced
- ½ cup mayo
- ¼ cup sour cream
- 1 tsp white distilled vinegar
- salt
- 6 oz. cheddar, cut into small cubes

Directions:

1. In a mixing bowl, combine the cheddar, broccoli, bacon, almonds, and onion.
2. Stir these ingredients thoroughly.
3. In another bowl, combine the sour cream, mayo, vinegar, and salt.
4. Stir the ingredients well and pour this mixture over your broccoli salad.

Nutritional Information per Serving:

Cal. 267 - Fats 20 g - Carbs 7 g - Prot. 12 g

FATTY BURGER BOMBS

Prep.: 15 min. | **Cook:** 15 min. | **Servings:** 20

Ingredients:

- 1-pound ground beef
- ½ tsp garlic powder
- Kosher salt and black pepper
- 1 oz. cold butter, cut into 20 pieces
- ½ block cheddar cheese, cut into 20 pieces

Directions:

1. Preheat the oven to 375°F.
2. In a separate bowl, the mix ground beef, garlic powder, salt, and pepper.
3. Use a mini muffin tin to form your bombs.
4. Put about 1 Tbsp. of beef into each muffin tin cup.
5. Make sure that you completely cover the bottom.
6. Add a piece of butter on top and put 1 Tbsp. of beef over the butter.
7. Place a piece of cheese on the top and put the remaining beef over the cheese.
8. Bake your bombs for about 15 minutes.

Nutritional Information per Serving:

Cal. 80 - Fats 7 g - Carbs 0 g - Prot. 5 g

AVOCADO TACO

Prep.: 10 min. | **Cook:** 15 min. | **Servings:** 6

Ingredients:

- 1-pound ground beef
- 3 avocados, halved
- 1 Tbsp. Chili powder
- ½ tsp salt
- ¾ tsp cumin
- ½ tsp oregano, dried
- ¼ tsp garlic powder
- ¼ tsp onion powder
- 8 Tbsp. tomato sauce
- 1 cup cheddar cheese, shredded
- ¼ cup cherry tomatoes, sliced
- ¼ cup lettuce, shredded

- ½ cup sour cream

Directions:

1. Pit halved avocados. Set aside.
2. Place the ground beef into a saucepan.
3. Cook over medium heat until it is browned.
4. Add the seasoning and tomato sauce.
5. Stir well and cook for about 4 minutes.
6. Load each avocado half with the beef.
7. Top with shredded cheese and lettuce, tomato slices, and sour cream.

Nutritional Information per Serving:

Cal. 278 - Fats 22 g - Carbs 2 g - Prot. 18 g

CHICKEN QUESADILLAS

Prep.: 10 min. | **Cook:** 15 min. | **Servings:** 2

Ingredients:

- 1½ cups Mozzarella cheese, shredded
- 1½ cups Cheddar cheese, shredded
- 1 cup chicken, cooked and shredded
- 1 bell pepper, sliced
- ¼ cup tomato, diced
- ⅛ cup green onion
- 1 Tbsp. extra-virgin olive oil

Directions:

1. Preheat the oven to 400°F.
2. Use parchment paper to cover a pizza pan.
3. Combine your cheeses and bake the cheese shell for about 5 minutes.
4. Put the chicken on one half of the cheese shell.
5. Add peppers, tomatoes, green onion and fold your shell in half over the fillings.
6. Return your folded cheese shell to the oven again for 4-5 minutes.

Nutritional Information per Serving:

Cal. 599 - Fats 40 g - Carbs 6.1 g - Prot. 52 g

SALMON SUSHI ROLLS

Prep.: 15 min. | **Cook:** 15 min. | **Servings:** 5 (4 pieces each)

Ingredients:

- 4 oz. smoked salmon
- ¼ red bell pepper, cut into matchstick pieces
- ½ cucumber, cut into matchstick pieces
- ½ avocado
- 20 seaweed sheets
- ½ cup Water

Directions:

1. Cut the salmon and avocado the same way that you cut the red pepper and cucumber.
2. Place seaweed snacks on a cutting board.
3. Put a cup of water nearby.
4. Wet your fingers with water and wet one edge of each seaweed sheet.
5. Put one piece of salmon, pepper, cucumber, and avocado on each seaweed snack and roll them up.

Nutritional Information per Serving:

Cal. 320 - Fats 20 g - Carbs 8 g - Prot. 24 g

MEDITERRANEAN SALAD WITH GRILLED CHICKEN

Prep.: 25 min. | **Cook:** 15 min. | **Servings:** 4

Ingredients:

- 4 romaine lettuce leaves, washed and dried
- 1 cucumber, diced
- 2 tomatoes, diced
- 1 red onion, sliced
- 1 avocado, sliced
- ⅓ cup Kalamata olives, pitted and chopped

- 2 Tbsp. olive oil
- ¼ cup lemon juice
- 2 Tbsp. water
- 2 Tbsp. red wine vinegar
- 2 Tbsp. parsley, chopped
- 2 Tbsp. basil, dried
- 2 Tbsp. garlic, chopped
- 1 tsp oregano, dried
- 1 tsp salt
- Black pepper, to taste
- 1-pound chicken fillets

Directions:

1. To make the marinade, mix the olive oil, lemon juice, water, red wine vinegar, parsley, basil, oregano, salt, and pepper. Divide the marinade into two halves.
2. Place the chicken into the marinade for 15-30 minutes.
3. In a separate bowl combine the lettuce leaves, cucumber, tomatoes, onion, avocado and olives. Stir well.
4. Pour 1 Tbsp. of oil into a pan and grill the chicken until it is browned on both sides. Slice your chicken and add it to the salad.
5. Sprinkle your salad with the remaining marinade.

Nutritional Information per Serving:

Cal. 336 - Fats 21 g - Carbs 13 g - Prot. 24 g

CREAMY CAULIFLOWER SOUP

Prep.: 10 min. | **Cook:** 40 min. | **Servings:** 5

Ingredients:

- 21 head cauliflower, cut into florets
- 3 Tbsp. olive oil
- ¾ tsp sea salt
- 4 cloves garlic
- 1 Tbsp. thyme, fresh
- 4 cups chicken broth

- 8 oz. cream cheese, cut into cubes
- ¼ tsp black pepper
- Green onion, chopped
- Parsley, chopped

Directions:

1. Preheat the oven to 425°F.
2. Place the cauliflower florets into a bowl.
3. 2 Tbsp. of olive oil over them and ¼ tsp of sea salt.
4. Bake for about 30 minutes in the oven.
5. Place the remaining olive oil in a pot, add the garlic and thyme and sauté for 1 minute.
6. Pour the chicken broth and baked cauliflower into the pot.
7. Boil for 5-10 minutes.
8. Add the cream cheese and mix the soup with an immersion blender.
9. Top with green onion and parsley.

Nutritional Information per Serving:

Cal. 286 - Fats 24 g - Carbs 12 g - Prot. 6 g

EGG DROP SOUP

Prep.: 10 min. | **Cook:** 20 min. | **Servings:** 6

Ingredients:

- 1 tbsp. olive oil
- 6 cups chicken broth, divided
- 1 tbsp. arrowroot powder
- Ground white pepper, to taste
- 1 tbsp. garlic, minced
- 2 organic eggs
- 1/3 cup fresh lemon juice
- ¼ cup scallion (green part), chopped

Directions:

1. In a large soup pan, heat the oil over medium-high heat and sauté garlic for about 1 minute.
2. Add 5½ cups of broth and bring to a boil over high heat.

3. Adjust the heat to medium and simmer for about 5 minutes.
4. Meanwhile, in a bowl, add eggs, arrowroot powder, lemon juice, white pepper, and remaining broth, and beat until well combined.
5. Slowly, add egg mixture in the pan, stirring continuously.
6. Simmer for about 5–6 minutes or until desired thickness of soup, stirring continuously.
7. Serve hot with the garnishing of scallion.

Nutritional Information per Serving:

Cal. 92 - Fats 5.3 g - Carbs 3.4 g - Prot. 7 g

BROCCOLI CHEESE SOUP

Prep.: 5 min. | **Cook:** 20 min. | **Servings:** 8

Ingredients:

- Broccoli (4 cups, chopped)
- Garlic (4 cloves, minced)
- Chicken broth (3.5 cups)
- Heavy cream (1 cup)
- Cheddar cheese (3 cups, shredded)

Directions:

1. Set a large greased saucepan with garlic over medium heat.
2. Sauté until fragrant (about a minute).
3. Add in your remaining ingredients except cheese, and switch to high heat.
4. Allow to come to a boil, then switch the heat to low and allow to simmer until broccoli becomes fork tender.
5. Gradually add cheese, while stirring, and continue to simmer until the cheese has been fully melted.
6. Serve immediately and enjoy!

Nutritional Information per Serving:

Cal. 266 - Fats 23 g - Carbs 2.6 g - Prot. 13 g

CREAMY TOMATO-BASIL SOUP

Prep.: 5 min. | **Cook:** 15 min. | **Servings:** 4

Ingredients:

- 2 ounces cream cheese
- 1 (14.5-ounce) can diced tomatoes
- ¼ cup chopped fresh basil leaves
- ¼ cup heavy (whipping) cream
- 4 tablespoons butter

Directions:

1. In a food processor, add the tomatoes with juices and pulse until smooth.
2. In a medium saucepan, add the tomatoes, heavy cream, cream cheese, and butter over medium heat and cook for 10 minutes, stirring often.
3. Stir in the basil, salt and pepper and cook for 5 minutes or until smooth.
4. Pour the soup into two bowls and serve.

Nutritional Information per Serving:

Cal. 239 - Fats 22 g - Carbs 9 g - Prot. 3 g

SPICY CAULIFLOWER SOUP

Prep.: 10 min. | **Cook:** 13 min. | **Servings:** 4

Ingredients:

- 1 1/2 cups water
- 1 cup carrot, sliced into 2-inch thick pieces
- 1 teaspoon salt
- 2 cup cauliflower florets, sliced into 3 to 4-inch chunks
- 1 cup (canned) tomatoes
- 1 onion (large) sliced into 2-inch thick pieces
- 1 teaspoon turmeric
- 1 to 1 1/2 teaspoons Sambhar powder

Directions:

1. Put all the ingredients in the inner pot; stir to mix well.
2. Secure the lid and place pressure valve to seal position.
3. Set to LOW PRESSURE for 3 minutes.
4. NPR for 10 minutes when the timer beeps and QPR; unlock the lid and open.
5. Stir to mix well.
6. Serve.

Nutritional Information per Serving:

Cal. 43 - Fats 0.3 g - Carbs 6.3 g - Prot. 2 g

CHEESE & BACON CAULIFLOWER SOUP

Prep.: 10 min. | **Cook:** 30 min. | **Servings:** 5

Ingredients:

- 1 cup celery
- 1 head cauliflower
- 1/2 stick butter
- 2 clove garlic (large)
- 3/4 cup cream (heavy)
- 1 cup cheddar cheese
- 1/2 cup parmesan, extra for garnish
- 1/3 up carrots
- 3 bacon slices
- 32 ounces chicken stock

Directions:

1. Chop 1/2 of the cauliflower; grate the other half.
2. Prepare the other veggies.
3. Set the IP to SAUTÉ.
4. Add the bacon; cook till crisped and remove.
5. Add the butter to the pot. Add the grated cauliflower.
6. Add the rest of the veggies; sauté for 5 minutes.
7. Add the cream; stir to mix.

8. Add the garlic, pepper, salt, and broth.
9. Secure the lid and place pressure valve to seal position.
10. Set to HIGH PRESSURE for 15 minutes.
11. NPR when the timer beeps; unlock the lid and open.
12. Stir in the cheeses till melted. Add the bacon.
13. Stir to mix.
14. Serve.

Nutritional Information per Serving:

Cal. 462 - Fats 37 g - Carbs 8 g - Prot. 22 g

BLACK SOYBEAN SOUP

Prep.: 10 min. | **Cook:** 40 min. | **Servings:** 4-6

Ingredients:

- 1 small red onion, diced
- 1 tablespoon cumin
- 1/2 teaspoon cayenne pepper
- 14 ounces dry black soybeans
- Avocado salsa, for garnish, optional
- 1 red pepper, diced
- 1/2 bunch cilantro leaves & stems, divided
- 2 tablespoons chili powder
- 3 cloves garlic, minced
- 3 cups vegetable broth, plus extra water

Directions:

1. Place the onion, garlic, and cilantro stems in the IP.
2. Add a splash of water.
3. Set the IP to SAUTE; cook for 2 to 3 minutes or till translucent.
4. Add the red pepper and spices; sauté for 1 to 2 minutes.
5. Add the soybeans and broth; stir to mix well.
6. Add enough water to cover the beans with 1-inch water.

7. Secure the lid and place pressure valve to seal position.
8. Set to MANUAL HIGH PRESSURE for 30 minutes.
9. QPR when the timer beeps; unlock the lid and open.
10. Puree all or only 1/2 of the soup using an immersion or regular blender.

Nutritional Information per Serving:

Cal. 174 - Fats 7.1 g - Carbs 8.6 g - Prot. 14.3 g

AVOCADO WITH BROCCOLI AND ZUCCHINI SALAD

Prep.: 10 min. | **Cook:** 10 min. | **Servings:** 4

Ingredients:

- 1 large zucchini, julienne
- 1/2 cup broccoli, cut into florets
- 2 avocados, sliced
- 2 cup goat cheese
- 1 tablespoon apple cider vinegar

Directions:

1. Combine zucchini, goat cheese, broccoli, and vinegar, then mix well.
2. Season to taste, and top with avocado slices.
3. Serve, and enjoy.

Nutritional Information per Serving:

Cal. 215 - Fats 17.6 g - Carbs 6.1 g - Prot. 9.8 g

CREAMY KALE SALAD

Prep.: 10 min. | **Cook:** 0 min. | **Servings:** 3

Ingredients:

- Kale (2 bunches)
- 1 cup sour cream
- 2 tablespoons sesame seeds oil
- 2 tbsp. lemon juice

Toppings

- Goat Cheese (6 oz.)

Directions:

1. Chop kale and wash kale then remove the ribs.
2. Transfer kale to a large bowl.
3. Add sour cream, and sesame seeds oil.
4. Season to taste and mix thoroughly.
5. Top with your goat cheese.
6. Serve and enjoy.

Nutritional Information per Serving:

Cal. 78 - Fats 6.4 g - Carbs 3.2 g - Prot. 1.1 g

CHEESY ROASTED BRUSSELS SPROUT SALAD

Prep.: 10 min. | **Cook:** 15min. | **Servings:** 2

Ingredients:

- Brussels sprouts (1 lb.)
- 1 tablespoon olive oil
- Feta cheese (1 cup, crumbled)
- Parmesan cheese (¼ cup, grated)
- Hazelnuts (¼ cup, whole, skins removed)

Directions:

1. Set your oven to preheat to 350°F.
2. Line a baking sheet with a silicone baking mat or parchment paper.
3. Trim the bottom and core from each Brussels sprout with a small knife.
4. Put the leaves in a medium bowl; you can use your hands to release all the leaves fully.
5. Toss the leaves with the olive oil and season with pink salt and pepper.
6. Add your leaves evenly in the bottom of your baking sheet.
7. Roast for 10 to 15 minutes, or until lightly browned and crisp.

8. Divide the roasted Brussels sprouts leaves between two bowls, top each with the shaved Parmesan cheese and hazelnuts, and serve.

Nutritional Information per Serving:

Cal. 287 - Fats 19 g - Carbs 9 g - Prot. 14 g

LETTUCE GROUND BEEF SALAD

Prep.: 10 min. | **Cook:** 5 min. | **Servings:** 2-3

Ingredients:

- ½ Cup of Grated Cheese
- 2 Cups of Chopped Lettuce
- 1 Medium Avocado
- ½ of a Medium lime
- ½ Cup of Sour Cream
- 2 Tbsp. of chopped Red Onion Chopped
- Sugar free salsa
- 1 lb. of beef mince
- ¼ tsp of garlic Powder
- ¼ tsp of dried Oregano
- ½ tsp of Paprika
- 1 and ½ tsp of ground cumin
- ¾ Cup of water

Directions:

1. Heat your Air Fryer to a temperature of about 390°F.
2. Place the meat, the seasoning and 2 tbsp. of water in your Air Fryer Pan.
3. Season the meat with 1 pinch of salt and 1 pinch of ground black pepper.
4. Place the Air Fryer pan in your Air Fryer and lock the lid.
5. Set the timer to about 5 minutes and set the temperature to 390°F.
6. When the timer beeps; turn off your Air Fryer.
7. Transfer the ground meat to a serving platter and cover with the chopped lettuce.
8. Season your salad with 1 pinch of salt and drizzle with olive oil.

9. Serve and enjoy your salad!

Nutritional Information per Serving:

Cal. 310 - Fats 18 g - Carbs 9 g - Prot. 23 g

SHRIMP AND AVOCADO LETTUCE CUPS

Prep.: 10 min. | **Cook:** 5 min. | **Servings:** 2

Ingredients:

- 1 tablespoon ghee
- ½ pound shrimp
- ½ cup halved grape tomatoes
- ½ avocado, sliced
- 4 butter lettuce leaves, rinsed and patted dry

Directions:

1. In a medium skillet over medium-high heat, heat the ghee.
2. Add the shrimp and cook.
3. Season with pink salt and pepper.
4. Shrimp are cooked when they turn pink and opaque.
5. Season the tomatoes and avocado with pink salt and pepper.
6. Divide the lettuce cups between two plates.
7. Fill each cup with shrimp, tomatoes, and avocado.
8. Drizzle the mayo sauce on top and serve.

Nutritional Information per Serving:

Cal. 326 - Fats 11 g - Carbs 7 g - Prot. 33 g

SALMON WRAPS

Prep.: 15 min. | **Cook:** 0 min. | **Servings:** 4

Ingredients:

- 4 Swiss chard leaves
- 4 tbsp. unsweetened coconut milk
- 4 scallions, chopped
- Salt and ground black pepper, to taste
- 1 cup cooked salmon
- 2 tbsp. fresh lemon juice
- 2 tbsp. fresh dill, chopped

Directions:

1. Arrange Swiss chard leaves onto a cutting board, face down.
2. Carefully, remove the bulk of each leaf, but not so much that the full leaf separates.
3. In a blender, add the coconut milk, lemon juice, scallions, dill, salt and black pepper and pulse until smooth.
4. In a small bowl, add the salmon and ½ of scallion sauce and mix well.
5. Arrange chard leaves onto serving plates.
6. Divide salmon mixture over the leaves evenly.
7. Serve immediately alongside with remaining sauce.

Nutritional Information per Serving:

Cal. 129 - Fats 7.4 g - Carbs 4.8 g - Prot. 12.8 g

CHEESY BUFFALO CHICKEN LETTUCE WRAPS

Prep.: 15 min. | **Cook:** 15 min. | **Servings:** 4

Ingredients:

- 1 cup chicken broth (low-sodium)
- 1-ounce cream cheese
- 1/2 cup cheese (cheddar), shredded
- 3/4 cup buffalo sauce
- Blue cheese, crumbled
- Preferred chicken seasoning to taste
- 1 green onion, chopped
- 1 tablespoon Greek yogurt (plain)
- 2 chicken breasts (skinless)
- 4 slices romaine lettuce
- Pepper & salt to taste

Directions:

1. Put the chicken and broth in the IP.
2. Secure the lid and place pressure valve to seal position.
3. Set to MANUAL HIGH PRESSURE for 10 minutes.
4. NPR for 10 minutes when the timer beeps and QPR; unlock the lid and open.
5. Transfer the chicken to a slicing board.
6. Shred using 2 forks or a knife.
7. Remove the cooking liquid from the pot.
8. Set the IP to SAUTÉ.
9. Add the shredded meat.
10. Add the cream cheese, buffalo sauce, cheddar, yogurt, pepper, salt, and chicken seasoning.
11. Stir to mix.
12. Cook for 2 to 3 minutes or till the cheese is melted.
13. Put the mixture on lettuce wraps.
14. Top with crumbled blue cheese and green onions.

Nutritional Information per Serving:

Cal. 215 - Fats 8.8 g - Carbs 2.3 g - Prot. 31.5 g

STUFFED AVOCADO

Prep.: 10 min. | **Cook:** 0 min. | **Servings:** 2

Ingredients:

- 1 large avocado, halved and pitted
- 3 tbsp. mayonnaise
- 2 tbsp. fresh lemon juice
- Salt and black pepper, to taste
- 1 (5-ounce) can water-packed tuna, drained and flaked
- 1 tbsp. onion, chopped finely

Directions:

1. Carefully, remove abut about 2–3 tablespoons of flesh from each avocado half.
2. Arrange the avocado halves onto a platter and drizzle each with 1 teaspoon of lemon juice.
3. Chop the avocado flesh and transfer into a bowl.
4. In the bowl of avocado flesh, add tuna, mayonnaise, onion, remaining lemon juice, salt, and black pepper, and stir to combine.
5. Divide the tuna mixture in both avocado halves evenly. Serve immediately.

Nutritional Information per Serving:

Cal. 396 - Fats 32.3 g - Carbs 8 g - Prot. 19.9 g

DINNER RECIPES

CRAB MELT

Prep.: 5 min. | **Cook:** 20 min. | **Servings:** 4

Ingredients:

- 2 zucchini
- A single tablespoon olive oil
- 3 ounces of stalks from celery
- 3/4 cup of mayo
- 12 ounces of crab meat
- A single red bell pepper
- 7 ounces of cheese (use shredded cheddar)
- A single tablespoon of Dijon mustard

Directions:

1. Preheat your oven to 450°F.
2. Slice your zucchini lengthwise.
3. Go for about a half-inch thick.
4. Add salt.
5. Let it sit for 15 minutes.
6. Pat it dry with a paper towel.
7. Place your slices on a baking sheet.
8. The baking sheet needs to be lined with parchment paper.
9. Brush olive oil on each side.
10. Finely chop the vegetables.
11. Mix with the other ingredients.
12. Apply mix to zucchini.
13. Bake for 20 minutes.
14. Your top will be golden brown.

Nutritional Information per Serving:

Cal. 542 - Fats 45 g - Carbs 7 g - Prot. 20 g

SPINACH FRITTATA

Prep.: 10 min. | **Cook:** 35 min. | **Servings:** 4

Ingredients:

- 5 ounces of diced bacon
- 2 tablespoons of butter
- 8 ounces of spinach that's fresh
- 8 eggs
- A single cup of heavy whipping cream
- 5 ounce of shredded cheese

Directions:

1. Preheat your oven to 350°F and grease a 9 by 9 baking dishes.
2. Fry your bacon on a heat medium until it is crispy.
3. Add your spinach and stir until it has wilted.
4. Remove pan from heat.
5. Place it to the side.
6. Whisk cream and eggs together and pour into the baking dish.
7. Add the spinach and bacon and pour the cheese on top.
8. Put in the middle of the oven.
9. Bake a half hour.
10. It should be set in the middle.
11. The color on top should be golden brown.

Nutritional Information per Serving:

Cal. 661 - Fats 59 g - Carbs 4 g - Prot. 27 g

HALLOUMI TIME

Prep.: 5 min. | **Cook:** 15 min. | **Servings:** 2

Ingredients:

- 3 ounces of halloumi cheese that have been diced
- 2 chopped scallions
- 4 ounces of diced bacon
- 2 tablespoons of olive oil
- 4 tablespoons of chopped fresh parsley
- 4 eggs
- Half a cup of pitted olives

Directions:

1. In a frying pan on medium-high heat, heat the oil.
2. Fry the scallions, cheese, and bacon until they are nicely browned.
3. Get a bowl and whisk your eggs and parsley together.
4. Pour the egg mix into the pan over the bacon.
5. Lower heat.
6. Add olives.
7. Stir for 2 minutes.

Nutritional Information per Serving:

Cal. 663 - Fats 59 g - Carbs 4 g - Prot. 28 g

POBLANO PEPPERS

Prep.: 5 min. | **Cook:** 15 min. | **Servings:** 2

Ingredients:

- A pound of grated cauliflower
- 3 ounces of butter
- 4 eggs
- 3 ounces of poblano peppers
- A single tablespoon of olive oil
- Half a cup of mayo

Directions:

1. Put your mayo in a bowl to the side.
2. Grate the cauliflower, including the stem.
3. Fry the cauliflower for 5 minutes in the butter.

4. Brush the oil on the peppers.
5. Fry them until you see the skin bubble a little.
6. Fry your eggs any way you like.
7. Servings with mayo.

Nutritional Information per Serving:

Cal. 898 - Fats 87 g - Carbs 9 g - Prot. 17 g

HASH BROWNS

Prep.: 20 min. | **Cook:** 10 min. | **Servings:** 4

Ingredients:

- 3 eggs
- A pound of cauliflower
- Half a grated yellow onion
- 4 ounces of butter

Directions:

1. Rinse the cauliflower.
2. Trim it.
3. Grate it using a food processor.
4. Add it to a bowl.
5. Add everything and mix.
6. Set aside 10 minutes.
7. Melt a right amount of butter on medium heat.
8. You need a larger skillet.
9. Place the mix in the pan and flatten.
10. Fry for 5 minutes on each side.
11. Don't burn it.

Nutritional Information per Serving:

Cal. 282 - Fats 26 g - Carbs 5 g - Prot. 7 g

SALAD WITH BUTTER

Prep.: 5 min. | **Cook:** 10 min. | **Servings:** 2

Ingredients:

- 10 ounces of goat cheese
- A quarter cup of pumpkin seeds
- 2 ounces of butter

- Tablespoons of balsamic vinegar
- 3 ounces of spinach (use baby spinach)

Directions:

1. Preheat oven to 400°F
2. Put goat cheese in a baking dish that is greased.
3. Bake 10 minutes.
4. Toast pumpkin seeds in a frying pan that is dry.
5. The temperature should be reasonably high.
6. They need some color, and they should start to pop.
7. Lower heat.
8. Add butter and simmer till it smells nutty and is golden brown.
9. Add vinegar and boil 3 minutes.
10. Turn off heat.
11. Spread the spinach on your plate and top with cheese and sauce.

Nutritional Information per Serving:

Cal. 824 - Fats 73 g - Carbs 3 g - Prot. 37 g

MUSHROOM OMELET

Prep.: 5 min. | **Cook:** 10 min. | **Servings:** 1

Ingredients:

- 4 sliced large mushrooms
- A quarter chopped yellow onion
- A single ounce of shredded cheese
- An ounce of butter
- 3 eggs

Directions:

1. Crack the eggs and whisk them.
2. When smooth and frothy, they are right.
3. Melt butter over medium heat in a frying pan.
4. Add onions and mushrooms and stir until they become tender.
5. Pour the egg mix in.
6. Surround the veggies.

7. When the omelet begins to get firm but is still a little raw on top, add cheese.
8. Carefully ease around the edges and fold in half.
9. When it's golden brown underneath (turning this color), remove and plate it.

Nutritional Information per Serving:

Cal. 517 - Fats 4 g - Carbs 5 g - Prot. 26 g

TUNA CASSEROLE

Prep.: 7 min. | **Cook:** 20 min. | **Servings:** 4

Ingredients:

- A single green bell pepper
- 5 ⅓ celery stalks
- 16 ounces of tuna in olive oil and drained
- A single yellow onion
- 2 ounces of butter
- A single cup of mayo
- 4 ounces of parmesan cheese freshly shredded
- A single teaspoon of chili flakes

Directions:

1. Preheat your oven to 400°F
2. Chop all of the bell peppers, onions, and celery finely before frying it in butter in a frying pan. They should be slightly soft.
3. Mix mayo and tuna with the flakes and cheese.
4. This should be done in a greased baking dish.
5. Add the veggies.
6. Stir.
7. Bake 20 minutes.
8. It should be golden brown.

Nutritional Information per Serving:

Cal. 653 - Fats 43 g - Prot. 23 g - Carbs 5 g

GOAT CHEESE FRITTATA

Prep.: 15 min. | **Cook:** 30 min. | **Servings:** 2

Ingredients:

- 4 ounces of goat cheese
- 5 ounces of mushrooms
- 3 ounces of fresh spinach
- 2 ounces of scallions
- 2 ounces of butter
- Half a dozen eggs

Directions:

1. Preheat your oven to 350°F
2. Crack the eggs and whisk before crumbling cheese in the mix.
3. Cut mushrooms into wedge shapes.
4. Chop up the scallions.
5. Melt the butter in a skillet that is oven proof and cook scallions and mushrooms over medium heat for 10 minutes. They will be golden brown (or should be).
6. Add spinach and sauté two minutes.
7. Pour egg mixture into the skillet.
8. Place in the oven uncovered and bake 20 minutes.
9. It should be golden brown in the center.

Nutritional Information per Serving:

Cal. 774 - Fats 67 g - Carbs 6 g - Prot. 35 g

KETO PASTA

Prep.: 5 min. | **Cook:** 1 minute | **Servings:** 1

Ingredients:

- A single large egg yolk
- A single cup of mozzarella cheese that is part-skim low moisture and shredded

Directions:

1. In a bowl safe for the microwave, you will need to microwave the cheese for 60 seconds.
2. Stir until it's totally melted.
3. Allow cooling for 60 seconds.
4. Add in yolk and stir. It should make a yellow dough.
5. Place it on a flat surface that has been lined with parchment paper.
6. Place another paper over the dough.
7. Get a rolling pin and roll dough.
8. Remove the top piece when the dough is an eighth of an inch thick.
9. Cut the dough into half-inch wide strips.
10. Put in the fridge for 6 hours.
11. Put pasta in a pot of boiling water to cook and do not add salt.
12. Cook for 60 seconds, don't cook too long.
13. Remove and run under cold water.
14. Separate the strands.

Nutritional Information per Serving:

Cal. 358 - Fats 22 g - Carbs 3 g - Prot. 33 g

MEATY SALAD

Prep.: 5 min. | **Cook:** 10 min. | **Servings:** 2

Ingredients:

- 3.5 ounces of salami slices
- 2 cups of spinach
- A single avocado large and diced
- 2 tablespoons of olive oil
- A single teaspoon of balsamic vinegar

Directions:

1. Toss it all together.

Nutritional Information per Serving:

Cal. 454 - Fats 42 g - Carbs 10 g - Prot. 9 g

Tomato Salad

Prep.: 10 min. | **Cook:** 5 min. | **Servings:** 2

Ingredients:

- A dozen small spear asparagus
- 4 raw cherry tomatoes
- A cup and a half of arugula
- A single tablespoon of olive oil
- A tablespoon of whole pieces' pine nuts
- A teaspoon of maple syrup
- Tablespoon balsamic vinegar
- 2 tablespoons soft goat cheese

Directions:

1. Cut the tough ends off asparagus and throw away.
2. Place the asparagus in a pan of boiling water and cook 3 minutes.
3. Put in a bowl of ice-cold water right away.
4. Chill for 60 seconds. Drain.
5. Put on a plate.
6. Slice your tomatoes in half, place on top of the greens. (Arugula and asparagus)
7. Toss to combine.
8. Add the nuts to a pan that's dry and on a low heat toast for 2 minutes until it is lightly golden.
9. Add the syrup and vinegar along with the olive oil to a bowl and whisk, so they combine.
10. Drizzle the dressing on top and crumble your cheese.
11. Sprinkle the nuts over the top.

Nutritional Information per Serving:

Cal. 234 - Fats 18 g - Carbs 7 g - Prot. 7 g

Lemon Butter Fish

Prep.: 10 min. | **Cook:** 20 min. | **Servings:** 6

Ingredients:

- 1 tbsp. lemon juice
- 4 tbsp. butter, unsalted
- Sea salt & pepper, to taste
- 2 tbsp. almond flour
- 2 tbsp. olive oil
- 2 tilapia fillets
- Sea salt & pepper, to taste

Directions:

1. Warm the butter in a small pan over medium heat.
2. Warm the butter until it's slightly browned.
3. Add the lemon juice, pepper, and salt and stir constantly.
4. Adjust seasoning to taste.
5. Set aside while you cook your fillets.
6. Rinse the fish fillets and pat them dry before sprinkling with salt and pepper.
7. Spread the flour on a plate or shallow dish and dredge the fillets, spreading the flour over the fillets as needed.
8. Heat a non-stick skillet over medium heat and warm the oil in it until it's shimmering.
9. Place the fillets in the pan and cook for about two minutes per side until golden and crisp on either side.
10. Remove the fish from the heat and place on the plate.
11. Drizzle the sauce over it and serve immediately!

Nutritional Information per Serving:

Cal. 393 - Fats 28 g - Carbs 3 g - Prot. 31 g

Chili Lime Cod

Prep.: 10 min. | **Cook:** 10 min. | **Servings:** 2

Ingredients:

- 1/3 c. coconut flour
- ½ tsp. cayenne pepper

- 1 egg, beaten
- 1 lime
- 1 tsp. crushed red pepper flakes
- 1 tsp. garlic powder
- 12 oz. cod fillets
- Sea salt & pepper, to taste

Directions:

1. Preheat the oven to 400°F and line a baking sheet with non-stick foil.
2. Place the flour in a shallow dish (a plate works fine) and drag the fillets of cod through the beaten egg.
3. Dredge the cod in the coconut flour, then lay on the baking sheet.
4. Sprinkle the tops of the fillets with the seasoning and lime juice.
5. Bake for 10 to 12 minutes until the fillets are flaky.
6. Serve immediately!

Nutritional Information per Serving:

Cal. 215 - Fats 5 g - Carbs 3 g - Prot. 37 g

LEMON GARLIC SHRIMP PASTA

Prep.: 10 min. | **Cook:** 10 min. | **Servings:** 4

Ingredients:

- ½ lemon, thinly sliced
- ½ tsp. paprika
- 1 lb. lg. shrimp, deveined & peeled
- 1 tsp. basil, fresh & chopped
- 14 oz. Miracle Noodle Angel Hair pasta
- 2 cloves garlic, minced
- 2 tbsp. butter
- 2 tbsp. extra virgin olive oil
- Sea salt & pepper, to taste

Directions:

1. Drain the packages of Miracle noodles and rinse them under cold running water.

2. Bring a pot of water to a boil and place the noodles in the boiling water for two minutes before pulling them back out again.
3. Place the boiled noodles in a hot pan over medium heat and allow the excess moisture to cook off of them.
4. Set aside.
5. Add the butter and olive oil to the pan, then add the garlic and stir.
6. Place the shrimp and the lemon slices in the pan and allow to cook until the shrimp is done, about three minutes per side.
7. Once the shrimp is done, add the salt, pepper, and paprika to the pan, then top with the noodles.
8. Toss to coat everything together, top with basil, and serve!

Nutritional Information per Serving:

Cal. 360 - Fats 21 g - Carbs 4 g - Prot. 36 g

ONE-PAN TEX MEX

Prep.: 5 min. | **Cook:** 10 min. | **Servings:** 4

Ingredients:

- 1/3 c. baby corn, canned
- 1/3 c. cilantro, chopped & separated
- ½ c. chicken stock
- ½ c. diced tomatoes & green chiles
- ½ tsp. garlic powder
- ½ tsp. oregano
- 1 tsp. cumin
- 2 c. cauliflower, riced
- 2 c. chicken breast, cooked & diced
- 2 c. Mexican cheese blend, shredded
- 2 tbsp. extra virgin olive oil
- 2 tsp. chili powder

Directions:

1. Slice baby corn into small pieces and set aside.

2. Press any liquid out of the riced cauliflower and set aside.
3. In a large pan over medium heat, warm your oil and sauté the cauliflower rice for about two minutes.
4. Add all ingredients except for the cheese and cilantro, and stir well to cook.
5. Stir in about half of the cilantro and allow the flavors to meld.
6. Stir about half the cheese into the mix and stir until melted and combined.
7. Serve and top with remaining cheese and cilantro for garnish!

Nutritional Information per Serving:

Cal. 345 - Fats 26 g - Carbs 7 g - Prot. 38 g

SPINACH ARTICHOKE-STUFFED CHICKEN BREASTS

Prep.: 15 min. | **Cook:** 15 min. | **Servings:** 6

Ingredients:

- ¼ c. Greek yogurt
- ¼ c. spinach, thawed & drained
- ½ c. artichoke hearts, thinly sliced
- ½ c. mozzarella cheese, shredded
- 1 ½ lbs. chicken breasts
- 2 tbsp. olive oil
- 4 oz. cream cheese
- Sea salt & pepper, to taste

Directions:

1. Pound the chicken breasts to a thickness of about one inch. Using a sharp knife, slice a "pocket" into the side of each.
2. This is where you will put the filling.
3. Sprinkle the breasts with salt and pepper and set aside.
4. In a medium bowl, combine cream cheese, yogurt, mozzarella, spinach, artichoke, salt, and pepper and mix completely.

5. A hand mixer may be the easiest way to combine all the ingredients thoroughly.
6. Spoon the mixture into each breast's pockets and set aside while you heat a large skillet over medium heat and warm the oil in it. If you have extra filling you can't fit into the breasts, set it aside until just before your chicken is done cooking.
7. Cook each breast for about eight minutes per side, then pull off the heat when it reaches an internal temperature of about 165°F.
8. Before you pull the chicken out of the pan, heat the remaining filling to warm it through and rid it of any cross-contamination from the chicken.
9. Once hot, top the chicken breasts with it.
10. Serve.

Nutritional Information per Serving:

Cal. 288 - Fats 17 g - Carbs 2 g - Prot. 28 g

CHICKEN PARMESAN

Prep.: 20 min. | **Cook:** 15 min. | **Servings:** 4

Ingredients:

- ¼ c. avocado oil
- ¼ c. almond flour
- ¼ c. parmesan cheese, grated
- ¾ c. marinara sauce, sugar-free
- ¾ c. mozzarella cheese, shredded
- 2 lg. eggs, beaten
- 2 tsp. Italian seasoning
- 3 oz. pork rinds, pulverized
- 4 lg. chicken breasts, boneless & skinless
- Sea salt & pepper, to taste

Directions:

1. Preheat the oven to 450°F and grease a baking dish.

2. Place the beaten egg into one shallow dish. Place the almond flour in another. In a third dish, combine the pork rinds, parmesan, and Italian seasoning and mix well.
3. Pat the chicken breasts dry and pound them down to about ½ thick.
4. Dredge the chicken in the almond flour, then coat in egg, then coat in crumb.
5. Heat a large sauté pan over medium-high heat and warm oil until shimmering.
6. Once the oil is hot, lay the breasts into the pan and not move them until they've had a chance to cook.
7. Cook for about two minutes, then flip as gently as possible (a fish spatula is perfect) then cook for two more. Remove the pan from the heat.
8. Place the breasts in the greased baking dish and top with marinara sauce and mozzarella cheese.
9. Bake for about 10 minutes.
10. Serve!

Nutritional Information per Serving:

Cal. 621 - Fats 34 g - Carbs 6 g - Prot. 67 g

BOLOGNESE SAUCE

Prep.: 15 min. | **Cook:** 45 min. | **Servings:** 10

Ingredients:

- ¼ c. dry white wine
- ¼ c. parsley, chopped
- ½ c. half & half
- 1 lg. white onion, diced
- 1 tbsp. butter, unsalted
- 2 lb. ground beef
- 2 med. carrots, diced
- 2 med. stalks, diced
- 3 bay leaves
- 4 oz. pancetta or bacon, chopped
- 56 oz. crushed tomatoes
- Sea salt & pepper, to taste

Directions:

1. Heat a large pot over medium heat and brown the bacon or pancetta for about eight minutes.
2. Add the butter into the pot and stir in the celery and carrots.
3. Cook until they're soft.
4. Add the ground meat to the pot, along with salt and pepper to taste.
5. Break the meat up into chunks as it browns.
6. Add the wine to the sauce and allow it to reduce for a few minutes.
7. Add the crushed tomatoes to the pot and stir completely, then add bay leaves, salt, pepper, and stir once more.
8. Cover and allow to simmer for twenty minutes.
9. Add the cream to the pot and pull the bay leaves out of the sauce.
10. Serve!

Nutritional Information per Serving:

Cal. 191 - Fats 9 g - Carbs 13 g - Prot. 12 g

SHEET PAN JALAPEÑO BURGERS

Prep.: 10 min. | **Cook:** 20 min. | **Servings:** 4

Ingredients:

- 24 oz. ground beef
- Sea salt & pepper, to taste
- ½ tsp. garlic powder
- 6 slices bacon, halved
- 1 med. onion, sliced into ¼ rounds
- 2 jalapeños, seeded & sliced
- 4 slices pepper jack cheese
- ¼ c. mayonnaise
- 1 tbsp. chili sauce
- ½ tsp. Worcestershire sauce
- 8 lg. leaves of Boston or butter lettuce
- 8 dill pickle chips

Directions:

1. Preheat the oven to 425°F and line a baking sheet with non-stick foil.
2. Mix the salt, pepper, and garlic into the ground beef and form 4 patties out of it.
3. Line the burgers, bacon slices, jalapeño slices, and onion rounds onto the baking sheet and bake for about 18 minutes.
4. Top each patty with a piece of cheese and set the oven to boil.
5. Broil for 2 minutes, then remove the pan from the oven.
6. Serve one patty with 3 pieces of bacon, jalapeño slices, onion rounds, and desired amount of sauce with 2 pickle chips and 2 pieces of lettuce.
7. Enjoy!

Nutritional Information per Serving:

Cal. 608 - Fats 46 g - Carbs 5 g - Prot. 42 g

GRILLED HERB GARLIC CHICKEN

Prep.: 5 min. | **Cook:** 10 min. | **Servings:** 4

Ingredients:

- 1 ¼ lbs. chicken breasts, boneless & skinless
- 1 tbsp. garlic & herb seasoning mix
- 2 tsp. extra virgin olive oil
- Sea salt & pepper, to taste

Directions:

1. Heat a grill pan or your grill.
2. Coat the chicken breasts in a little bit of olive oil and then sprinkle the seasoning mixture onto them, rubbing it in.
3. Cook the chicken for about eight minutes per side and ensure the chicken has reached an internal temperature of 330°F.
4. Serve hot with your favorite sides!

Nutritional Information per Serving:

Cal. 187 - Fats 6 g - Carbs 1 g - Prot. 32 g

BLACKENED SALMON WITH AVOCADO SALSA

Prep.: 5 min. | **Cook:** 10 min. | **Servings:** 4

Ingredients:

- 1 tbsp. extra virgin olive oil
- 4 filets of salmon (about 6 oz. each)
- 4 tsp. Cajun seasoning
- 2 med. avocados, diced
- 1 c. cucumber, diced
- ¼ c. red onion, diced
- 1 tbsp. parsley, chopped
- 1 tbsp. lime juice
- Sea salt & pepper, to taste

Directions:

1. Heat a skillet over medium-high heat and warm the oil in it.
2. Rub the Cajun seasoning into the fillets, then lay them into the bottom of the skillet once it's hot enough.
3. Cook until a dark crust forms, then flip and repeat.
4. In a medium mixing bowl, combine all the ingredients for the salsa and set aside.
5. Plate the fillets and top with ¼ of the salsa Servings.
6. Enjoy!

Nutritional Information per Serving:

Cal. 445 - Fats 31 g - Carbs 10 g - Prot. 35 g

KETO ROMANIAN NOODLES

Prep.: 15 Min. | **Cook:** 10 Min. | **Servings:** 2

Ingredients:

- 3 eggs
- 2Tbsp. cream cheese
- 1Tbsp. mayo
- 2Tbsp. psyllium husks
- ¼ tsp salt

Directions:

1. First of all, preheat oven at 350 degrees.
2. In a blender add cream cheese, mayo, eggs, salt and psyllium husks and make a fine blend until the mixture got smooth.
3. Let the mixture set aside for 10 minutes.
4. Now set the silicone mat over the baking try, pour the egg mixture over the matt or spread it with a spatula.
5. Let it bake for 8 to 10 minutes or until cooked.
6. Let it cool down for at least 15 minutes.
7. After that, cut it and roll out with the help of knife.
8. Enjoy the keto noodles with pasta sauce.

Nutritional Information per Serving:

Cal. 223 - Fats 18 g - Carbs 7 g - Prot. 10 g

LOW CARB CAULIFLOWER COTTAGE PIE

Prep.: 15 min. | **Cook:** 55 min. | **Servings:** 5

Ingredients:

- 500 g lamb
- 1 onion, chopped
- Salt to taste
- Black pepper to taste
- 1 garlic clove
- 1 tsp coconut flour
- ½ tbsp. rosemary, chopped

For topping:

- 1 cauliflower
- 1 garlic clove
- 1 cup sour cream
- 55 g butter
- Salt & pepper to taste
- Cheddar cheese as desired

Directions:

1. Take a pan and heat it over the medium flame, add oil and heat then add lamb and cook for 10 to 12 minutes or until turn brown. Dish out and set aside.
2. Now add onion, salt, pepper in a pan and sauté for few minutes. Add garlic and cook for 1 more minute.
3. Add rosemary and stir well. Add the cooked lamb meat and mix them to combine well. Now set the oven at 400°F for preheating.
4. Meanwhile, cook the cauliflower over the steam for 6 to 8 minutes or until soft and tender. When cooked, drain them and transfer into a blender.
5. Add garlic, cream cheese, butter, salt, pepper, and blend them until smooth.
6. Now set the small pie pan. Add the lamb meat mixture and set well. Over it, pour the topping mixture and cover it well with the cheddar cheese.
7. Bake it for 20 to 25 minutes or until cooked or the cheese is melted.

Nutritional Information per Serving:

Cal. 382 - Fats 25 g - Carbs 5 g - Prot. 27 g

EASY CASHEW CHICKEN

Prep.: 15 min. | **Cook:** 10 min. | **Servings:** 3

Ingredients:

- 3 chicken thigh
- 2Tbsp. coconut oil
- ¼ cup Raw cashew
- ½ bell pepper, green
- ½ tsp ginger
- 1 ½ liquid aminos
- ½ tbsp. chili garlic sauce
- 1Tbsp. garlic
- 1Tbsp. sesame oil
- 1Tbsp. sesame seeds
- 1 tbsp. green onion

- ¼ white onion
- Salt & pepper to taste

Directions:

1. Take a pan and heat it over the medium flame.
2. Add cashews and roast them for 7 to 8 minutes or until turn light brown.
3. Set them aside.
4. Cut the chicken, bell peppers, and onion with the sharp knife into large chunks.
5. Add the coconut oil into pan and heat over the high flame.
6. Add chicken and cook it for 5 minutes.
7. When chicken fully cooked add bell pepper, onion, garlic, chili sauce, ginger, salt and pepper and cook for 3 to 4 minutes.
8. After that add liquid aminos and cashews and cook them on high flame until got the sticky consistency.
9. Pour it into a serving bowl and add sesame seed and sesame oil before serving.

Nutritional Information per Serving:

Cal. 333 - Fats 24 g - Carbs 8 g - Prot. 22 g

KETO CREAMY CHICKEN &MUSHROOM

Prep.: 10 min. | **Cook:** 20 min. | **Servings:** 4

Ingredients:

- 1 lb. chicken tenderloin
- ½ lb. mushrooms, sliced
- 2 tbsp. butter
- 2 tbsp. olive oil
- 2 garlic clove, chopped
- ¼ cup fresh parsley
- 2 tbsp. thyme leaves
- Salt & pepper to taste
- ½ cup chicken stock
- 1/2 cup heavy cream

- ¼ cup sour cream

Directions:

1. Take a pan and heat butter over the low medium flame.
2. Add chicken tenderloin and stir until golden brown on each side.
3. Pour it onto a plate and set aside.
4. In same pan, add more butter, olive oil, and mushrooms and cook them for 3 to 4 minutes or until brown and crispy.
5. Add the garlic, parsley, thyme leaves, chicken stock and cook well for 5 minutes.
6. When start simmer add cream, sour cream and cook over the low flame that mixture start simmer or turn thick.
7. Now toss the chicken tenderloin in to the mixture and cook for 5 to 6 minutes. Serve with parsley and thyme garnishing.

Nutritional Information per Serving:

Cal. 400 - Fats 29 g - Carbs 5 g - Prot. 27 g

CHICKEN WITH PABLANO PEPPERS &CREAM

Prep.: 10 min. | **Cook:** 20 min. | **Servings:** 4

Ingredients:

- 1 ¼ lb. chicken boneless
- 1 garlic clove
- 2 poblano pepper
- 1 cup heavy cream
- 3 ½ oz. onion
- 1/8 tsp cumin, dried
- 1Tbsp. olive oil
- Salt & pepper to taste

Directions:

1. First of all, roast the poblano pepper by placing it on a grill and cover it with the

plastic wrap for 5 to 10 minutes before cutting and peeling.

2. After that, heat the non-stick skillet with the oil.
3. Meanwhile, take boneless chicken, toss it with olive oil, and sprinkle some salt and pepper and cook over the skillet for 4 to 6 minutes from each side.
4. Wrap the chicken with the foil to keep it warm and soft.
5. For the sauce take a pan, heat oil and add onion to cook for 2 minutes.
6. Now add cream, poblano peppers, and cumin or cook until the cream gets thick and becomes required consistency.
7. Add some salt and pepper to taste and serve the chicken with the cream sauce.

Nutritional Information per Serving:

Cal. 484 - Fats 42 g - Carbs 6 g - Prot. 20 g

SHRIMP SHEET PAN FAJITAS

Prep.: 5 min. | **Cook:** 15 min. | **Servings:** 4

Ingredients:

- 1 ½ lb. shrimp, peeled
- 1 red bell pepper
- 1 orange bell pepper
- ½ cup poblano, sliced
- 1 cup red onion, sliced
- 1 ½ tbsp. olive oil
- 2tbsp. chili powder
- 1tsp cumin
- ½ tsp coriander
- ½ cup sour cream
- ½ tsp cilantro
- ½ tbsp. jalapeno, chopped
- 1Tbsp. lime & lime zest
- 1 garlic clove
- 2 corn tortillas
- ½ cup cilantro leaves
- 1 lime wedges

Directions:

1. Preheat the oven at 400°F. Set the baking pan with the foil and set shrimps over the tray. Add bell peppers, poblano, onion, olive oil, chili, cumin, and coriander, salt and toss them well over shrimp.
2. Now put it into oven and bake for 10 to 12 minutes. After that, remove the shrimp into a plate and cover to keep them warm.
3. Set the vegetables into the oven for 3 to 4 more minutes.
4. In a small bowl, add sour cream, cilantro, jalapeno, lime zest and juice, and mix with garlic. Add some salt to taste and combine well until smooth and creamy.
5. Now warm the tortillas and set the shrimp and vegetables over the tortillas and top it with sour cream and cilantro leaves. Serve them with lime wedges.

Nutritional Information per Serving:

Cal. 446 - Fats 20 g - Carbs 45 g - Prot. 26 g

CHEESY BRUSSELS SPROUTS

Prep.: 5 min. | **Cook:** 22 min. | **Servings:** 8

Ingredients:

- 3 Tbsp. butter
- ¼ cup shallot, sliced
- 2 garlic clove
- 32 oz. Brussels sprout
- Salt to taste
- Black pepper as per taste
- Paprika as desired
- ¾ cup heavy cream
- ¾ cup cheddar cheese
- ½ cup Gruyere cheese
- 6 strips of bacon
- Parsley for garnish

Directions:

1. Preheat oven at 375°F.
2. In a pan, heat butter over a medium flame and add Brussel sprouts, shallots, garlic, salt, pepper and paprika.
3. Cook them for 5 to 8 minutes, continuously stirring the whole time.
4. Pour the mixture into a baking pan, pour heavy cream, and mix well.
5. Sprinkle some cheddar cheese and gruyere cheese over the Brussel sprout and top it with the bacon slices.
6. Bake them for 12 minutes or until cheese melts and turns light brown.
7. Sprinkle some pepper, parsley leaves and serve.

Nutritional Information per Serving:

Cal. 311 - Fats 25 g - Carbs 11 g - Prot. 11 g

KETO ALFREDO ZOODLES

Prep.: 10 min. | **Cook:** 15 min. | **Servings:** 4

Ingredients:

- 3 zucchini
- 1 tsp butter
- 2 garlic cloves
- ¼ tsp nutmeg
- ½ cup almond milk
- 1/3 cup heavy cream
- ¾ cup parmesan cheese
- 1 Tbsp. arrowroot powder
- Black pepper to taste

Directions:

1. To make the zucchini noodles, use the fine cutter or a peeler.
2. Take a pan and heat it over the medium flame with butter.
3. Add garlic and fry it for a minute or until soft.
4. Now set over a low flame and pour almond milk, heavy cream, and nutmeg

and mix well. Let it simmer for few minutes.
5. In a small bowl, add arrowroot powder and water to make a smooth mixture. Pour this mixture into the almond milk mixture, gradually stirring.
6. Now add the parmesan cheese and black pepper and whisk well.
7. Cook it until cheese melts and achieves the required sauce consistency.
8. Meanwhile, fry the zucchini noodles over a medium high flame in a pan for 3 to 4 minutes or until soft.
9. Mix the noodles with sauce and garnish with parsley and serve.

Nutritional Information per Serving:

Cal. 209 - Fats 16 g - Carbs 9 g - Prot. 11 g

CREAM OF MUSHROOM SOUP WITH TARRAGON OIL

Prep.: 30 min. | **Cook:** 35 min. | **Servings:** 4

Ingredients:

- 40 g butter
- 1 onion
- 1 garlic clove
- 200 g mushrooms
- 200 g Swiss mushroom
- 2 potato
- 3 cup chicken stock
- ¼ cup tarragon leaves
- ¼ cup olive oil
- ¾ cup cream
- 50 g mushroom for garnishing

Directions:

1. Take a pan and heat butter over the medium flame. Add onion and garlic or sauté for 2 to 3 minutes.
2. Now add mushroom and cook for 4 to 5 minutes or until tender.

3. After that add the chicken stock, potato and ½ cup water to cook.
4. Cook the mixture for at least 20 minutes or until potatoes tender and stock turn half.
5. Set it aside to cool down for few minutes.
6. Meanwhile add the tarragon leaves in a blender with olive oil and make a smooth mixture. Take it out after blend.
7. Now, pour the soup into the blender and make a smooth blend. Put the cream soup and tarragon mixture together and cook over medium flame over 5 minutes.
8. Simultaneously, in a pan, fry the chopped mushroom on medium flame until turn brown.
9. Pour the soup into the bowl add the fried mushrooms as a topping and some tarragon leaves right before serving.

Nutritional Information per Serving:

Cal. 1847 - Fats 41 g - Carbs 4 g - Prot. 6 g

CHICKEN BACON RANCH CASSEROLE

Prep.: 15 min. | **Cook:** 35 min. | **Servings:** 8

Ingredients:

- ¼ c. yellow onion, diced
- ½ c. sour cream
- 1 ½ lbs. chicken thighs, cooked & chopped
- 1 c. mayonnaise
- 1 lb. broccoli, chopped
- 1 tbsp. parsley, fresh & chopped
- 2 c. cheddar cheese, shredded & divided
- 2 tsp. garlic powder
- 4 slices bacon, chopped
- 8 oz. cream cheese, softened
- Sea salt & pepper to taste

Directions:

1. Preheat the oven to 350°F and grease a baking dish with non-stick spray or your preferred fat source.
2. Add about an inch of water to a large saucepan and lower a steamer insert or metal strainer into it.
3. Toss the broccoli into the steamer and bring the water to a boil for about eight minutes or until tender.
4. Drain the excess moisture from the broccoli and set aside.
5. In a large mixing bowl, combine mayonnaise, sour cream, and cream cheese.
6. Into the mixing bowl, add the parsley, salt, pepper, and garlic powder. Using a whisk or a fork, beat the mixture until smooth.
7. Toss the broccoli, chicken, onion, half of the chopped bacon and 1 ½ cups of shredded cheese to the bowl and fold it in completely.
8. Pour the mixture into the baking dish and press into an even layer.
9. Top the casserole with the remaining cheese and bacon.
10. Bake for 35 minutes or until the cheese is bubbling.

Nutritional Information per Serving:

Cal. 504 - Fats 42 g - Carbs 5 g - Prot. 38 g

LETTUCE-WRAPPED SLOPPY JOES

Prep.: 15 min. | **Cook:** 20 min. | **Servings:** 4

Ingredients:

- ¼ c. tomato paste
- ½ head Boston or butter lettuce, leaves pulled off
- 1 lb. ground beef
- ¾ c. beef broth
- 1 med. stalk celery, diced
- 1 sm. yellow onion, diced

- 1 tsp. Dijon mustard
- 2 cloves garlic, minced
- 2 tbsp. erythritol sweetener or comparable amount of desired sweetener
- 2 tsp. Worcestershire sauce
- Sea salt & pepper

Directions:

1. Heat a large skillet with olive oil over medium heat until the oil is hot.
2. Stir celery, garlic, and onion into the skillet and cook for about six minutes or until tender.
3. Add the remaining ingredients (except the lettuce) to the skillet, stir well to combine.
4. Reduce the heat to low and simmer for about 20 minutes to allow the sauce to thicken.
5. Spoon the mixture into the lettuce wraps and serve!
6. TIP: Top with a little bit of shredded Monterey Jack cheese!

Nutritional Information per Serving:

Cal. 240 - Fats 7 g - Carbs 4 g - Prot. 36 g

SPICY LIME WINGS

Prep.: 5 min. | **Cook:** 35 min. | **Servings:** 6

Ingredients:

For the Wings:

- ¼ c. sugar-free maple syrup
- ½ c. Thai chili paste
- 2 tbsp. rice wine vinegar
- 2 tbsp. soy sauce
- 3 lb. chicken wings, separated at the joints

For the Dipping Sauce:

- ¼ c. mayonnaise
- 1 tbsp. lime juice, fresh

- 1/3 c. Greek yogurt, full fat, plain
- Sea salt & pepper to taste

Directions:

1. In a large mixing bowl, combine the maple syrup, chili paste, vinegar, and soy sauce and whisk thoroughly.
2. Toss the wings in the cause and cover.
3. Chill for about 3 hours to allow the marinade to work.
4. Preheat the oven to 400°F and line a baking sheet with non-stick foil.
5. Place the wings onto the baking sheet, ensuring that they're not overlapping.
6. Bake the wings for 30 minutes, flipping them over halfway through to ensure even cooking and crispness.
7. Place wings under the broiler for 3-4 minutes until they're nice and brown.
8. In a small bowl, whisk together the ingredients for the dipping sauce.
9. Serve the wings hot with chilled dipping sauce!

Nutritional Information per Serving:

Cal. 240 - Fats 7 g - Carbs 4 g - Prot. 36 g

CHILI DOG CASSEROLE

Prep.: 15 min. | **Cook:** 50 min. | **Servings:** 8

Ingredients:

- ½ tsp. celery salt
- 1 c. cheddar cheese, shredded
- 1 c. low-carb tomato sauce
- 1 c. water
- 1 lb. ground beef
- 1 sm. red bell pepper, diced
- 1 sm. yellow onion, diced
- 1 tbsp. chili powder
- 1 tsp. cumin, ground
- 1 tsp. Worcestershire sauce
- 2 cloves garlic, minced
- 2 tbsp. tomato paste
- 8 hotdogs, halved lengthwise

- Sea salt & pepper to taste

Directions:

1. Preheat the oven to 400°F and grease a baking dish with non-stick spray or your preferred fat source.
2. Layer the hotdog halves along the bottom of the baking dish and set it aside.
3. In a large skillet over medium heat, let the oil heat up.
4. Once the oil is hot, combine peppers, onions, ground beef, and garlic. Cook until the beef is browned and make sure to break the beef into small chunks.
5. Pour tomato sauce, Worcestershire sauce, tomato paste, seasonings and water. Mix thoroughly and allow all ingredients to incorporate completely.
6. Bring the mixture to a boil and drop the heat to low. Simmer for about 30 minutes until the mixture gains a bit of thickness.
7. Spoon the chili onto the hotdogs in the baking dish and top with cheese.
8. Bake for about 20 minutes, or until warmed through and the cheese on top is bubbling to your preference. Let cool for about ten minutes before cutting.

Nutritional Information per Serving:

Cal. 365 - Fats 27 g - Carbs 4 g - Prot. 24 g

CHEESY MEATBALL BAKE

Prep.: 15 min. | **Cook:** 45 min. | **Servings:** 8

Ingredients:

- ½ c. parmesan cheese, grated
- 1 c. low-carb tomato sauce
- 1 c. mozzarella cheese, shredded
- 1 c. zucchini, shredded & pressed
- 1 lb. ground beef
- 1 lb. ground sausage
- 1 lg. egg

- 1 tbsp. garlic, minced
- 1 tsp. oregano, dried
- 2 c. provolone cheese, shredded
- 2 tsp. basil, dried
- Sea salt & pepper to taste

Directions:

1. Preheat the oven to 400°F and grease a baking dish with non-stick spray or your preferred fat source.
2. Place shredded zucchini into a kitchen towel or paper towel and press all the excess moisture from it.
3. In a large mixing bowl, combine zucchini, ground beef, ground sausage, egg, seasonings, mozzarella, and parmesan. Mix until completely combined.
4. Out of the mixture, make 32 meatballs and arrange them in one even layer in the baking dish.
5. Pour the tomato sauce into the baking dish, over the meatballs, and sprinkle the top's provolone cheese.
6. Place in the oven to bake for 30 minutes.
7. Drain the excess liquid from the baking dish and return to oven.
8. Bake for another 10 to 15 minutes, or until cheese is bubbly and brown.
9. Serve hot!

Nutritional Information per Serving:

Cal. 515 - Fats 38 g - Carbs 2 g - Prot. 39 g

CINNAMON PORK CHOPS

Prep.: 5 min. | **Cook:** 10 min. | **Servings:** 4

Ingredients:

- ¼ tsp. black pepper, ground
- ¼ tsp. nutmeg
- ½ tsp. salt
- 1 pinch cloves, ground
- 1 tbsp. apple cider vinegar

- 1 tbsp. erythritol or comparable measure of your preferred sweetener
- 1 tsp. cinnamon
- 2 tbsp. coconut oil
- 4 pork chops, boneless

Directions:

1. In a medium skillet over medium heat, warm the coconut oil.
2. Use salt and pepper to season either side of the pork chops, then add them to the heated pan.
3. In a small bowl, combine the sweetener, cinnamon, cloves, nutmeg, and vinegar.
4. Flip the pork chops after about five minutes, then drizzle the spice mixture over them.
5. Let those heat until fully cooked, about another four minutes.
6. Remove the pan's chops and place them with any remaining drippings in the pan drizzled on top.
7. TIP: Goes great with a side of mashed cauliflower or a bright side salad!

Nutritional Information per Serving:

Cal. 193 - Fats 11 g - Carbs 4 g - Prot. 23 g

CREAMED SPINACH

Prep.: 5 min. | **Cook:** 10 min. | **Servings:** 4

Ingredients:

- ¼ c. parmesan cheese, grated
- ¼ tsp. basil, dried
- ¼ tsp. oregano, dried
- ½ c. heavy cream
- 10 oz. spinach, fresh & chopped
- 2 tbsp. butter
- 3 cloves garlic, minced
- 3 oz. cream cheese, softened
- Sea salt & pepper

Directions:

1. Warm a large saucepan over medium heat and melt the butter in the pan.
2. Stir the garlic into the butter and allow to become fragrant.
3. Stir spinach into the pan and allow to wilt for about three to four minutes.
4. Stir heavy cream, salt, pepper, oregano, cream cheese, and basil into the pan until thoroughly combined.
5. Allow to cook for up to five minutes while the cream cheese melts, stirring constantly.
6. Sprinkle with parmesan cheese and serve!

Nutritional Information per Serving:

Cal. 220 - Fats 20.5 g - Carbs 3 g - Prot. 6.5 g

KETO FISH STICKS

Prep.: 10 min. | **Cook:** 15 min | **Servings:** 4

Ingredients:

- 1 ½ tbsp. coconut flour
- 1 lg. egg, beaten
- 1 tsp. water
- 12 oz. cod fillets, fresh & sliced into one-ounce strips
- 3 ½ oz. pork rinds

Directions:

1. Preheat the oven to 400°F and line a baking sheet with non-stick foil.
2. Slice fish into one-ounce strips and season to taste with salt and pepper.
3. Dredge the strips of fish into the coconut flour and coat evenly.
4. Crush the pork rinds into a coarse powder with either a rolling pin or a food processor, then pour into a shallow dish.
5. Beat the egg with the water in a shallow dish.

6. Coat each stick in the egg mixture, then in the pork rinds, ensuring that every stick's entire surface is coated completely.
7. Place each stick onto the baking sheet in an even layer.
8. Bake for 12 to 15 minutes or until golden brown and cooked through.
9. Serve hot!
10. TIP: Try mixing a little bit of horseradish and mayonnaise for a zesty dipping sauce!

Nutritional Information per Serving:

Cal. 270 - Fats 11.5 g - Carbs 1 g - Prot. 38 g

PARMESAN-CRUSTED COD

Prep.: 10 min | **Cook:** 15 min | **Servings:** 4

Ingredients:

- ¼ c. butter, melted
- ¾ c. parmesan cheese, grated
- 1 ½ lbs. cod fillets
- 1 tbsp. lemon zest, fresh
- 1 tbsp. parsley, fresh & chopped
- 1 tsp. paprika
- 2 cloves garlic, minced

Directions:

1. Preheat the oven to 400°F and place parchment paper inside baking sheet.
2. In a shallow dish, combine the melted butter and the garlic.
3. In another dish, combine paprika and parmesan, stir to combine.
4. Coat each filet in the melted butter mixture, then dredge in the parmesan.
5. Place each fillet on the baking dish and sprinkle with parsley and lemon zest,
6. Bake for about 15 minutes or until golden brown and cooked through.
7. Serve hot!
8. TIP: Try mixing a little bit of horseradish and mayonnaise together for a zesty dipping sauce!

Nutritional Information per Serving:

Cal. 320 - Fats 17.5 g - Carbs 1 g - Prot. 36 g

VEGETARIAN RECIPES

ZUCCHINI CAULIFLOWER FRITTERS

Prep.: 5 min. | **Cook:** 15 min. | **Servings:** 2

Ingredients:

- ¼ head of cauliflower, chopped (roughly 1 ½ cups)
- 1 tablespoon coconut oil
- 1/8 cup coconut flour
- 1 medium zucchini; grated
- Black pepper and sea salt to taste

Directions:

1. Steam the cauliflower until just fork tender, for 3 to 5 minutes.
2. Add cauliflower to your food processor and process on high power until broken down into very small chunks (ensure it's not mashed).
3. Squeeze the moisture as much as possible from the grated veggies using a nut milk bag or dishtowel.
4. Transfer to a large bowl along with the grated zucchini and add flour coconut flour followed by pepper, salt and any seasonings you desire; combine well.
5. Make 4 small-sized patties from the mixture.
6. Now, over moderate heat in a large pan; heat 1 tablespoon of coconut oil.
7. Work in batches and cook the fritters for 2 to 3 minutes per side.
8. The cooked fritters can be served with some dipping sauce of your choice on side.

Nutritional Information per Serving:

Cal. 112 - Fats 8 g - Carbs 5.6 g - Prot. 2.1 g

EGGLESS SALAD

Prep.: 5 min. | **Cook:** 5 min. | **Servings:** 4

Ingredients:

- 1 stalk celery, chopped
- Vegan mayonnaise, as required
- 1 pound extra firm tofu
- 2 tablespoons onions, minced
- Pepper and salt to taste

Directions:

1. Mash the tofu into a chunky texture, just like an egg salad.
2. Add mayonnaise until you get your desired consistency.
3. Add in the leftover ingredients; stir well.
4. Serve on keto pitas or keto bread, with vegetables and enjoy.

Nutritional Information per Serving:

Cal. 117 - Fats 7.8 - Carbs 2.8 g - Prot. 16 g

MOUTH-WATERING GUACAMOLE

Prep.: 5 min. | **Cook:** 0 min. | **Servings:** 6

Ingredients:

- 3 avocados, pitted
- ¼ cup cilantro, freshly chopped, plus more for garnish

- Juice of 2 limes
- ½ teaspoon kosher salt
- 1 small jalapeño, minced
- ½ small white onion, finely chopped

Directions:

1. Combine avocados with cilantro, lime juice, jalapeño, onion and salt in a large-sized mixing bowl; mix well.
2. Give the ingredients a good stir and then, slowly turn the bowl; running a fork through the avocados.
3. Once you get your desired level of consistency, immediately season it with more salt, if required.
4. Just before serving; feel free to garnish your recipe with more of fresh cilantro.

Nutritional Information per Serving:

Cal. 165 - Fat 15 g - Carbs 9.5 g - Prot. 2.1 g

ROASTED GREEN BEANS

Prep.: 5 min. | **Cook:** 30 min. | **Servings:** 4

Ingredients:

- 3 cups green beans, raw, trimmed
- 1 tablespoon Italian seasoning
- 2 tablespoons olive oil
- Ground black pepper and kosher salt to taste
- 4 tablespoons pumpkin seeds

Directions:

1. Combine green beans with olive oil and seasonings in a large bowl; toss to coat. Spread them out on a roasting pan or cookie sheet, preferably large-sized.
2. Roast in the oven for 20 minutes at 400°F.
3. Remove; give everything a good stir.
4. Place the cookie sheet again into the oven and roast for 10 more minutes.
5. Remove.

6. Sprinkle pumpkin seeds, serve warm and enjoy.

Nutritional Information per Serving:

Cal. 155 - Fats 12 g - Carbs 8.7 g - Prot. 6.4 g

FRIED TOFU

Prep.: 10 min. | **Cook:** 6 min. | **Servings:** 4

Ingredients:

- 1 teaspoon seasoning
- 3 tablespoons tamari or soya sauce
- 1 package extra firm tofu (350 g)
- ¼ cup Nutritional yeast
- 1 tablespoon olive oil

Directions:

1. Lightly coat a large, non-stick pan with some oil.
2. Put soy sauce (tamari) in a medium sized mixing bowl.
3. Mix the spices together with the yeast in a separate bowl.
4. Slice the tofu into slices, approximately ¼.
5. Dip the tofu pieces in the tamari and then into the yeast mixture.
6. Fry until golden, for 2 to 3 minutes; flip and let the other side become brown for 2 to 3 more minutes.
7. If required, add a bit of oil.

Nutritional Information per Serving:

Cal. 139 - Fats 8.6 - Carbs 5.1 g - Prot. 12.1 g

CURRY ROASTED CAULIFLOWER

Prep.: 5 min. | **Cook:** 15 min. | **Servings:** 2

Ingredients:

- 1/2-pound cauliflower, approximately a large head; remove the outer leaves, cut into half and then cut out and discard

the core; cutting it further into bite-sized pieces
- 2 tablespoons nuts; any of your favorites
- 1 ½ teaspoon curry powder
- 1 tablespoon plus 1 teaspoon extra-virgin olive oil
- 2 teaspoons lemon juice, fresh
- 1 teaspoon kosher salt

Directions:

1. Preheat your oven to 425°F.
2. Toss the cauliflower pieces with olive oil in a large bowl until evenly coated. Sprinkle with curry powder and salt.
3. Give everything a good toss until nicely coated.
4. Spread them out on a large-sized rimmed baking sheet, preferably in an even layer and transfer them to the preheated oven.
5. Roast for 8 to 10 minutes, until the bottom is starting to turn brown.
6. Turn them over and continue to roast for 5 to 7 more minutes, until fork-tender.
7. Place them to the bowl again
8. Toss with the freshly squeezed lemon juice and your favorite nuts.
9. Serve immediately and enjoy.

Nutritional Information per Serving:

Cal. 188 - Fats 16.7 g - Carbs 8.1 g - Prot. 6.3 g

ROASTED BRUSSELS SPROUTS WITH PECANS AND ALMOND BUTTER

Prep.: 5 min. | **Cook:** 35 min. | **Servings:** 4

Ingredients:

- 1 pound Brussels sprouts, fresh; ends trimmed
- ¼ cup almond butter
- 2 tablespoons olive oil
- ½ cup pecans, chopped or to taste
- Fresh ground black pepper and salt to taste

Directions:

1. Using a pastry brush; lightly coat a large-sized roasting pan with 1 tablespoon olive oil and preheat your oven to 350°F in advance.
2. Cut each Brussels sprout lengthwise into halves or fourths.
3. Chop the pecans using a sharp knife and measure the desired amount out.
4. Put the chopped pecans and Brussels sprouts into a large-sized plastic bowl and toss with 1 tablespoon olive oil.
5. Generously season with fresh ground black pepper and salt to taste.
6. Arrange the pecans and Brussels sprouts in a single layer on roasting pan.
7. Roast in the preheated oven until the sprouts begin to brown on the edges and are fork-tender, for 30 to 35 minutes, stirring several times during the cooking process.
8. Just before serving, toss the cooked pecans and Brussels sprouts with almond butter.
9. Serve hot and enjoy.

Nutritional Information per Serving:

Cal. 175 - Fats 23.5 g - Carbs 11 g - Prot. 7.6 g

SPINACH SOUP

Prep.: 10 min. | **Cook:** 15 min. | **Servings:** 8

Ingredients:

- Butter – 2 tbsp.
- Spinach – 20 ounces, chopped
- Garlic – 1 tsp. minced
- Salt and ground black pepper to taste
- Chicken stock – 45 ounces
- Ground nutmeg – ½ tsp.

- Heavy cream – 2 cups
- Onion – 1, chopped

Directions:

1. Heat a saucepan and melt the butter.
2. Add onion, and stir-fry for 4 minutes.
3. Add garlic, and stir-fry for 1 minute.
4. Add spinach and stock, and stir-fry for 5 minutes. Remove from heat.
5. Blend soup with a hand mixer and heat the soup again.
6. Add salt, pepper, and nutmeg, cream, stir, and cook for 5 minutes.
7. Serve.

Nutritional Information per Serving:

Cal. 158 - Fats 14 g - Carbs 5.4 g - Prot. 3.3 g

ASPARAGUS FRITTATA

Prep.: 10 min. | **Cook:** 15 min. | **Servings:** 4

Ingredients:

- Onion – ¼ cup, chopped
- A drizzle of olive oil
- Asparagus spears – 1-pound, cut into 1-inch pieces
- Salt and ground black pepper to taste
- Eggs – 4, whisked
- Cheddar cheese – 1 cup, grated

Directions:

1. Heat a pan with oil over medium heat.
2. Add onions, and stir-fry for 3 minutes.
3. Add asparagus and stir-fry for 6 minutes.
4. Add eggs and stir-fry for 3 minutes.
5. Add salt, pepper, and sprinkle with cheese.
6. Place in the oven and broil for 3 minutes.
7. Divide frittata on plates and serve.

Nutritional Information per Serving:

Cal. 202 - Fats 13 g - Carbs 5.8 g - Prot. 15 g

BELL PEPPERS SOUP

Prep.: 10 min. | **Cook:** 15 min. | **Servings:** 6

Ingredients:

- Roasted bell peppers – 12, seeded and chopped
- Olive oil – 2 tbsp. - Garlic – 2 cloves, minced - Vegetable stock – 30 ounces
- Salt and black pepper to taste - Water - 6 ounces
- Heavy cream – 2/3 cup
- Onion – 1, chopped
- Parmesan cheese – ¼ cup, grated
- Celery stalks – 2, chopped

Directions:

1. Heat a saucepan with oil over medium heat.
2. Add onion, garlic, celery, salt, and pepper.
3. Stir-fry for 8 minutes.
4. Add water, bell peppers, stock, stir, and bring to a boil.
5. Cover, lower heat, and simmer for 5 minutes.
6. Remove from heat and blend with a hand mixer.
7. Then adjust seasoning, and add cream.
8. Stir and bring to a boil.
9. Remove from the heat and serve on bowls.
10. Sprinkle with Parmesan and serve.

Nutritional Information per Serving:

Cal. 155 - Fats 12 g - Carbs 8.6 g - Prot. 4.7 g

RADISH HASH BROWNS

Prep.: 10 min. | **Cook:** 10 min. | **Servings:** 4

Ingredients:

- ½ tsp. onion powder
- 1 pound, radishes shredded
- ½ tsp. garlic powder
- Salt and ground black pepper to taste
- 4 Eggs
- 1/3 cup parmesan cheese grated

Directions:

1. In a bowl, mix radishes, with salt, pepper, onion, garlic powder, eggs, Parmesan cheese, and mix well.
2. Spread on a lined baking sheet.
3. Place in an oven at 375°F and bake for 10 minutes.
4. Serve.

Nutritional Information per Serving:

Cal. 104 - Fats 6 g - Carbs 4.5 g - Prot. 8.6 g

CELERY SOUP

Prep.: 10 min. | **Cook:** 30 min. | **Servings:** 6

Ingredients:

- Celery – 1 bunch, chopped
- Onion – 1, chopped
- Green onion – 1 bunch, chopped
- Garlic cloves – 4, minced
- Salt and ground black pepper to taste
- Parsley – 1 fresh bunch, chopped
- Fresh mint bunches – 2, chopped
- Persian lemons – 3 dried, pricked with a fork
- Water – 2 cups
- Olive oil – 4 Tbsp.

Directions:

1. Heat a saucepan with oil over medium heat.
2. Add onion, garlic, and green onions.
3. Stir and cook for 6 minutes.

4. Add Persian lemons, celery, salt, pepper, water, stir, cover pan, and simmer on medium heat for 20 minutes.
5. Add parsley and mint, stir, and cook for 10 minutes.
6. Blend with a hand mixer and serve.

Nutritional Information per Serving:

Cal. 100 - Fats 9.5 g - Carbs 4.4 g - Prot. 1 g

SPRING GREENS SOUP

Prep.: 10 min. | **Cook:** 30 min. | **Servings:** 4

Ingredients:

- Mustard greens – 2 cups, chopped
- Collard greens – 2 cups, chopped
- Vegetable stock – 4 cups
- Onion – 1, chopped
- Salt and ground black pepper to taste
- Coconut aminos – 2 Tbsp.
- Fresh ginger – 2 tsp. grated

Directions:

1. Put the stock into a saucepan and bring to a simmer over medium heat.
2. Add ginger, coconut aminos, salt, pepper, onion, mustard, and collard greens. Stir, cover, and cook for 30 minutes.
3. Remove from the heat.
4. Blend the soup with a hand mixer.
5. Serve.

Nutritional Information per Serving:

Cal. 35 - Fats 1 g - Carbs 7 g - Prot. 2 g

ALFALFA SPROUTS SALAD

Prep.: 10 min. | **Cook:** 10 min. | **Servings:** 4

Ingredients:

- Dark sesame oil – 1 ½ tsp.
- Alfalfa sprouts – 4 cups

- Salt and ground black pepper to taste
- Grapeseed oil – 1 ½ tsp.
- Coconut yogurt – ¼ cup

Directions:

1. In a bowl, mix sprouts with yogurt, grape seed oil, sesame oil, salt, and pepper. Toss to coat and serve.

Nutritional Information per Serving:

Cal. 83 - Fats 7.6 g - Carbs 3.4 g - Prot. 1.6 g

EGGPLANT STEW

Prep.: 10 min. | **Cook:** 30 min. | **Servings:** 4

Ingredients:

- Onion – 1, chopped
- Garlic – 2 cloves, chopped
- Fresh parsley – 1 bunch, chopped
- Salt and black pepper to taste
- Dried oregano – 1 tsp.
- Eggplants – 2, cut into chunks
- Olive oil – 2 Tbsp.
- Capers – 2 Tbsp. chopped
- Green olives – 12, pitted and sliced
- Tomatoes – 5, chopped
- Herb vinegar – 3 Tbsp.

Directions:

1. In a saucepan, heat oil over medium heat.
2. Add oregano, eggplant, salt, pepper, and stir-fry for 5 minutes.
3. Add parsley, onion, garlic, and stir-fry for 4 minutes.
4. Add tomatoes, vinegar, olives, capers, and stir-fry for 15 minutes.
5. Adjust seasoning and stir.
6. Serve.

Nutritional Information per Serving:

Cal. 280 - Fats 17 g - Carbs 8.4 g - Prot. 5 g

ZUCCHINI SALAD

Prep.: 10 min. | **Cook:** 10 min. | Servings 6

Ingredients:

- 2 pounds' zucchini
- 2 tbsp. butter or olive oil
- 3 oz. celery stalks, finely sliced
- 2 oz. chopped scallions
- 1 cup mayonnaise
- 2 pounds' zucchini
- 2 tbsp. butter or olive oil
- 3 oz. celery stalks, finely sliced
- 2 oz. chopped scallions
- 1 cup mayonnaise
- 2 tbsp. fresh chives, finely chopped
- ½ tablespoons Dijon Mustard
- Sea Salt
- Pepper

Directions:

1. Peel and cut the zucchini into pieces that are about half an inch thick. Use a spoon to remove the seeds.
2. Place in a colander and add salt. Leave for 5 – 10 minutes and then cautiously press out the water.
3. Fry the cubes in butter for a couple of minutes over medium heat. They should not brown, just slightly soften.
4. Set aside to cool.
5. Mix the other ingredients in a large bowl and add the zucchini once it's cool.
6. Tip: You can prepare the salad 1-2 days ahead of time; the flavors only enhance with time. You can also add a chopped hard- boiled egg.

Nutritional Information per Serving:

Cal. 312 - Fats 32 g - Carbs 4 g - Prot. 3 g

LOADED BAKED CAULIFLOWER

Prep.: 10 min. | **Cook:** 30 min. | Servings 2

Ingredients:

- 4 ounces bacon
- 1-pound cauliflower
- 2/3 cup sour cream
- ½ pound cheddar cheese, shredded
- 2 tbsp. chives, finely chopped
- 1 tsp garlic powder
- Sea salt
- Freshly ground pepper

Directions:

1. Preheat oven to 350°F.
2. Chop the bacon into small pieces.
3. Fry until crispy in a hot frying pan.
4. Reserve the fat for serving.
5. Break the cauliflower into florets.
6. Boil until soft in lightly salted water. Drain completely.
7. Chop the cauliflower roughly. Add sour cream and garlic powder.
8. Combine well with ¾ of the cheese and most of the finely chopped chives.
9. Salt and pepper
10. Place in a baking dish and top with the rest of the cheese.
11. Bake in the oven for 10 – 15 minutes or until the cheese has melted.
12. Top with the bacon, the rest of the chives and the bacon fat.
13. Enjoy.

Nutritional Information per Serving:

Cal. 614 - Fats 49 g - Carbs 10 g - Prot. 30 g

CABBAGE HASH BROWNS

Prep.: 10 min. | **Cook:** 12 min. | **Servings:** 2

Ingredients:

- 1 ½ cup shredded cabbage

- 2 slices of bacon
- 1/2 tsp garlic powder
- 1 egg
- 1 tbsp. coconut oil
- ½ tsp salt
- 1/8 tsp ground black pepper

Directions:

1. Crack the egg in a bowl, add garlic powder, black pepper, and salt, whisk well, add cabbage, and toss until well mixed and shape the mixture into four patties.
2. Take a large skillet pan, place it over medium heat, add oil and when hot, add patties in it and cook for 3 minutes per side until golden brown.
3. Transfer hash browns to a plate, then add bacon into the pan and cook for 5 minutes until crispy.
4. Serve hash browns with bacon.

Nutritional Information per Serving:

Cal. 336 - Fats 29.5 g - Carbs 1 g - Prot. 16 g

CAULIFLOWER HASH BROWNS

Prep.: 10 min. | **Cook:** 18 min. | **Servings:** 2

Ingredients:

- ¾ cup grated cauliflower
- 2 slices of bacon
- 1/2 tsp garlic powder
- 1 large egg white
- Seasoning:
- 1 tbsp. coconut oil
- ½ tsp salt
- 1/8 tsp ground black pepper

Directions:

1. Place grated cauliflower in a heatproof bowl, cover with plastic wrap, poke some holes in it with a fork and then microwave for 3 minutes until tender.

2. Let steamed cauliflower cool for 10 minutes, then wrap in a cheesecloth and squeeze well to drain moisture as much as possible.
3. Crack the egg in a bowl, add garlic powder, black pepper, and salt, whisk well, then add cauliflower and toss until well mixed and sticky mixture comes together.
4. Take a large skillet pan, place it over medium heat, add oil and when hot, drop cauliflower mixture on it, press lightly to form hash brown patties, and cook for 3 to 4 minutes per side until browned.
5. Transfer hash browns to a plate, then add bacon into the pan and cook for 5 minutes until crispy.
6. Serve hash browns with bacon.

Nutritional Information per Serving:

Cal. 347 - Fats 31 g - Carbs 1.2 g - Prot. 15.6 g

ASPARAGUS, WITH BACON AND EGGS

Prep.: 5 min. | **Cook:** 12 min. | **Servings:** 2

Ingredients:

- 4 oz. asparagus
- 2 slices of bacon, diced
- 1 egg
- Seasoning:
- ¼ tsp salt
- 1/8 tsp ground black pepper

Directions:

1. Take a skillet pan, place it over medium heat, add bacon, and cook for 4 minutes until crispy.
2. Transfer cooked bacon to a plate, add asparagus into the pan and cook for 5 minutes until tender-crisp.
3. Crack the egg over the cooked asparagus, season with salt and black

pepper, switch heat to medium-low level and cook for 2 minutes until the egg white has set.
4. Chop the cooked bacon slices, sprinkle over egg and asparagus and serve.

Nutritional Information per Serving:

Cal. 179 - Fats 15.3 g - Carbs 0.7 g - Prot. 9 g

BELL PEPPER EGGS

Prep.: 10 min. | **Cook:** 4 minutes | Serving: 2

Ingredients:

- 1 green bell pepper
- 2 eggs
- 1 tsp coconut oil
- ¼ tsp salt
- ¼ tsp ground black pepper

Directions:

1. Prepare pepper rings, and for this, cut out two slices from the pepper, about ¼-inch, and reserve remaining bell pepper for later use.
2. Take a skillet pan, place it over medium heat, grease it with oil, place pepper rings in it, and then crack an egg into each ring.
3. Season eggs with salt and black pepper, cook for 4 minutes, or until eggs have cooked to the desired level.
4. Transfer eggs to a plate and serve.

Nutritional Information per Serving:

Cal. 110 - Fats 8 g - Carbs 1.7 g - Prot. 7.2 g

OMELET-STUFFED PEPPERS

Prep.: 5 min. | **Cook:** 20 min. | **Servings:** 2

Ingredients:

- 1 large green bell pepper, halved, cored
- 2 eggs

- 2 slices of bacon, chopped, cooked
- 2 tbsp. grated parmesan cheese
- 1/3 tsp salt
- ¼ tsp ground black pepper

Directions:

1. Turn on the oven, then set it to 400°F, and let preheat.
2. Then take a baking dish, pour in 1 tbsp. water, place bell pepper halved in it, cut-side up, and bake for 5 minutes.
3. Meanwhile, crack eggs in a bowl, add chopped bacon and cheese, season with salt and black pepper, and whisk until combined.
4. After 5 minutes of baking time, remove baking dish from the oven, evenly fill the peppers with egg mixture and continue baking for 15 to 20 minutes until eggs have set.
5. Serve.

Nutritional Information per Serving:

Cal. 428 - Fats 35 g - Carbs 2.8 g - Prot. 23 g

CAULIFLOWER WITH ARTICHOKES PIZZA

Prep.: 10 min. | **Cook:** 30 min. | **Servings:** 1

Ingredients:

- 4.25 ounces (120 g) grated cauliflower
- 2 ounces (57 g) canned artichokes, cut into wedges
- 4.25 ounces (120 g) shredded cheese
- 2 eggs, beaten
- ½ teaspoons salt
- 2 tablespoons tomato sauce
- 2 ounces (57 g) shredded cheese
- 2 ounces (57 g) mozzarella cheese
- 1 thinly sliced garlic clove
- 1 tablespoon dried oregano

Directions:

1. Start by preheating the oven to 350°F.
2. In a bowl, add the cauliflower, shredded cheese, eggs and salt.
3. Stir them properly.
4. Using a spatula, spread the mixture in a thin layer on a baking sheet lined with a parchment paper, approximately 11-inch in diameter.
5. Arrange the baking sheet in the oven and bake for 20 minutes or until they turn into a nice color.
6. Remove the baking sheet from your oven, spread with tomato sauce, then top with the cheese, garlic and artichokes. Sprinkle with oregano.
7. Increase the temperature of the oven to 420°F.
8. Put the baking sheet back to the oven and bake the pizza for an extra 10 minutes.
9. Transfer the cooked pizza to a serving platter.
10. Allow to cool for a few minutes before serving

Nutritional Information per Serving:

Cal. 1010 - Fats 74 g - Carbs 13 g - Prot. 68 g

CHILI CABBAGE WEDGES

Prep.: 5 min. | **Cook:** 20 min. | **Servings:** 4

Ingredients:

- 1 medium head cabbage
- 1 teaspoon chili powder
- Pepper and salt
- ¼ cup olive oil

Directions:

1. Start by preheating the oven to 400°F.
2. Divide the cabbage into wedges then spread them out on to a baking sheet.
3. Add the chili powder, pepper and salt to season.

4. Sprinkle the olive oil on the cabbage and mix properly.
5. Put them in the oven.
6. Bake for about 20 minutes or until the wedges turn to a nice color.
7. Transfer to four serving bowls.
8. Allow to cool for a few minutes before serving.

Nutritional Information per Serving:

Cal. 108 - Fats 10 g - Carbs 3 g - Prot. 1.5 g

CAULIFLOWER, LEEKS AND BROCCOLI

Prep.: 5 min. | **Cook:** 15 min. | **Servings:** 4

Ingredients:

- 8 ounces cauliflower, chopped in bite-sized pieces
- 3 ounces leeks, chopped in bite-sized pieces
- 1 pound broccoli, chopped in bite-sized pieces
- 3 ounces butter
- 5 ounces shredded cheese
- ½ cup fresh thyme
- 4 tablespoons sour cream
- Pepper and salt to taste

Directions:

1. In a skillet over medium-high heat, add butter and heat to melt.
2. Add the leeks, broccoli and cauliflower.
3. Fry the vegetables until they become golden brown.
4. Add the cheese, thyme and sour cream.
5. Stir well until the cheese melts.
6. Add pepper and salt for seasoning.
7. Transfer them to a platter.
8. Allow to cool for a few minutes before serving

Nutritional Information per Serving:

Cal. 368 - Fats 32 g - Carbs 9.3 g - Prot. 14.2 g

LOW-CARB CHEESY OMELET

Prep.: 5 min. | **Cook:** 10 min. | **Servings:** 2

Ingredients:

- 6 eggs
- 7 ounces shredded Cheddar cheese
- Salt and ground black pepper, to taste
- 3 ounces butter

Directions:

1. In a bowl, whisk all the eggs until they are frothy and smooth.
2. Add half of the Cheddar and blend well.
3. Add the pepper and salt to season.
4. In a frying pan, melt the butter over medium-high heat, then pour the egg mixture and cook for a few minutes until you see the eggs at the edges of the pan beginning to set.
5. Reduce the heat to low as you continue cooking the mixture for 3 minutes until it is almost cooked.
6. Flip the omelet halfway through the cooking time.
7. Scatter the remaining cheese on top and cook for another 1 to 2 minutes until the cheese melts.
8. Fold your omelet and serve while warm.

Nutritional Information per Serving:

Cal. 899 - Fats 79 g - Carbs 5 g - Prot. 39.2 g

ROASTED GREEN BEANS WITH PARMESAN

Prep.: 10 min. | **Cook:** 20 min. | **Servings:** 4

Ingredients:

- 1 pound fresh green beans
- 1 egg

- ½ teaspoon salt
- ¼ teaspoon pepper
- 2 tablespoons olive oil
- 1 teaspoon onion powder
- 1 ounce grated Parmesan cheese

Directions:

1. Start by preheating the oven to 400°F.
2. In a bowl, whisk the egg, salt, pepper, oil and the onion powder.
3. Add the green beans, then toss to coat well.
4. Drain the excess liquid, then arrange the green beans in a baking sheet lined with parchment paper.
5. Sprinkle with Parmesan cheese.
6. Bake in the oven for about 20 minutes until the beans change to a nice color.
7. Transfer to four serving plates.
8. Allow to cool for a few minutes before serving.

Nutritional Information per Serving:

Cal. 143 - Fats 11 g - Carbs 5.8 g - Prot. 6.2 g

ROASTED SPICY BRUSSELS SPROUTS

Prep.: 5 min. | **Cook:** 16 min. | **Servings:** 4

Ingredients:

- 1 pound whole Brussels sprouts
- 2 tablespoons olive oil
- 1 onion, chopped
- ½ teaspoon ground black pepper
- 1 teaspoon salt
- ½ cup vegetable broth

Directions:

1. Select the 'Sauté' function on your instant pot.
2. Coat the instant pot with the olive oil.
3. Add the onions and cook for 2 minutes until they turn translucent.

4. Add the Brussels sprouts then cook them for an extra 1 minute.
5. Sprinkle with pepper and salt.
6. Pour the vegetable broth over the Brussels sprouts.
7. Close the lid of the instant pot.
8. Select the high-pressure function then set the timer to 3 minutes.
9. Allow about 15 minutes for pressure to build-up.
10. Release the pressure using the quick-release procedure for about 5 minutes then unlock and take the lid off.
11. Transfer to four serving bowls.
12. Allow to cool for a few minutes before serving.

Nutritional Information per Serving:

Cal. 123 - Fats 7.1 g - Carbs 13.6 g - Prot. 4.3 g

SPICY DEVILED EGGS IN CURRY PASTE

Prep.: 10 min. | **Cook:** 10 min. | **Servings:** 6

Ingredients:

- 6 eggs
- 3 cups water
- 1 tablespoon red curry paste
- ½ cup keto-friendly mayonnaise
- ¼ teaspoon salt
- ½ tablespoon poppy seeds

Directions:

1. In a pot of cold water.
2. Boil the eggs for 7 minutes until well done.
3. Reduce the heat to low and allow the eggs to simmer for 8 minutes.
4. Cool them instantly in ice-cold water.
5. Peel the eggs then divide the eggs into halves after cutting off both ends of the eggs.
6. Scoop the egg yolks out and place in a bowl.

7. Arrange the egg whites on a plate and place in the refrigerator.
8. Mix the egg yolks, curry paste, and mayonnaise to form a smooth batter.
9. Add salt to season.
10. Remove egg whites from the refrigerator and top with the batter evenly.
11. Sprinkle the poppy seeds as toppings.
12. Transfer to six serving plates and serve.

Nutritional Information per Serving:

Cal. 202 - Fats 20 g - Carbs 2 g - Prot. 6.2 g

SPICY HASH BROWNS WITH CAULIFLOWER

Prep.: 10 min. | **Cook:** 30 min. | **Servings:** 4

Ingredients:

- 3 eggs
- 1 pound rinsed, trimmed and grated cauliflower
- ½ grated yellow onion
- 2 pinches pepper
- 1 teaspoon salt
- 4 ounces butter

Directions:

1. In a bowl, whisk together the eggs, cauliflower, onion, pepper and salt. Set the mixture aside for about 10 minutes.
2. Place a skillet over medium-high heat and melt the butter.
3. Make the pancakes: Using ¼ cup measure, put scoops of the cauliflower mixture in a frying pan as you flatten them to about 4-inch (10 cm) in diameter.
4. Fry each side of the pancakes for about 5 minutes as you keep adjusting the heat to ensure that the pancakes do not burn.
5. Place the first batch of the pancakes (about 4) in the oven.

6. Keep the first batch of pancakes warm over low heat.
7. Repeat with the remaining cauliflower mixture.
8. Transfer them to four serving plates.
9. Allow to cool for a few minutes before serving.

Nutritional Information per Serving:

Cal. 281 - Fats 28 g - Carbs 4.3 g - Prot. 6.5 g

SWEET CREAMY CAULIFLOWER

Prep.: 15 min. | **Cook:** 30 min. | **Servings:** 6

Ingredients:

- 1 large head cauliflower, cut into bite-sized pieces
- 1 cup shredded mozzarella cheese
- ½ cup keto-friendly mayonnaise
- ½ cup sour cream
- 3 tablespoons chopped fresh chives
- ¼ cup bacon bits
- 1 cup shredded sharp Cheddar cheese

Directions:

1. Start by preheating the oven to 425°F.
2. Put a steamer insert into your saucepan then fill the saucepan with water up to a level slightly above the bottom of the steamer. Boil the water.
3. Add the cauliflower to the steamer.
4. Cover the lid and steam for 10 minutes or until tender.
5. Drain and cool for 10 minutes
6. In a large bowl, mix the mozzarella cheese, mayonnaise, sour cream, chives, and half of the bacon bits.
7. Add the cauliflower and stir to combine well.
8. Pour the mixture into a baking dish.
9. Sprinkle with the Cheddar cheese and remaining bits of the bacon.

10. Place in the oven and bake for about 20 minutes or until golden brown and all the cheese melts.
11. Transfer to six serving plates.
12. Allow to cool for a few minutes before serving.

Nutritional Information per Serving:

Cal. 366 - Fats 30.1 g - Carbs 9.5 g - Prot. 15.7 g

TASTY ROASTED BUFFALO CAULIFLOWER

Prep.: 10 min. | **Cook:** 40 min. | **Servings:** 4

Ingredients:

- ⅓ cup Buffalo wing sauce
- 1 tablespoon butter
- 2 tablespoons extra-virgin olive oil
- 1 head cauliflower, broken into small florets
- ¼ cup grated Parmesan cheese

Directions:

1. Adjust the temperature of your oven to 375°F.
2. In a microwave-safe bowl, add the Buffalo sauce, butter, and olive oil.
3. For about 1 minute, melt the butter in microwave.
4. Stir the mixture to combine.
5. Add the cauliflower florets and toss to coat.
6. Arrange the well-coated cauliflower on a baking sheet.
7. Place in the oven and bake for about 30 minutes.
8. Top with the Parmesan cheese.
9. Resume the baking until they are slightly toasted for an additional 10 minutes.
10. Remove from the oven.
11. Allow to cool before serving.

Nutritional Information per Serving:

Cal. 165 - Fats 11.8 g - Carbs 9 g - Prot. 5.6 g

GRAIN-FREE CREAMY NOODLES

Prep.: 15 min. | **Cook:** 10 min. | **Servings:** 4

Ingredients:

- 1¼ C. heavy whipping cream
- ¼ C. mayonnaise
- Salt and freshly ground black pepper, to taste
- 30 oz. zucchini, spiralized with blade C
- 4 organic egg yolks
- 3 oz. Parmesan cheese, grated
- 2 tbsp. fresh parsley, chopped
- 2 tbsp. butter, melted

Directions:

1. In a pan, add the heavy cream and bring to a boil.
2. Reduce the heat to low and cook until reduced.
3. Add the mayonnaise, salt and black pepper and cook until mixture is warm enough.
4. Add the zucchini noodles and gently, stir to combine.
5. Immediately, remove from the heat.
6. Place the zucchini noodles mixture onto 4 serving plates evenly and immediately, top with the egg yolks, followed by the parmesan and parsley.
7. Drizzle with hot melted butter and serve.

Nutritional Information per Serving:

Cal. 427 - Fats 39.1 g - Carbs 9 g - Prot. 13 g

MEAT-FREE ZOODLES STROGANOFF

Prep.: 20 min. | **Cook:** 12 min. | **Servings:** 5

Ingredients:

For Mushroom Sauce:

- 1½ tbsp. butter
- 1 large garlic clove, minced
- 1¼ C. fresh button mushrooms, sliced
- ¼ C. homemade vegetable broth
- ¼ C. cream
- Salt and freshly ground black pepper, to taste

For Zucchini Noodles:

- 3 large zucchinis, spiralized with blade C
- ¼ C. fresh parsley leaves, chopped

Directions:

1. For mushroom sauce: In a large skillet, melt the butter over medium heat and sauté the garlic for about 1 minute.
2. Stir in the mushrooms and cook for about 6-8 minutes.
3. Stir in the broth and cook for about 2 minutes, stirring continuously.
4. Stir in the cream, salt and black pepper and cook for about 1 minute.
5. Meanwhile, for the zucchini noodles: in a large pan of the boiling water, add the zucchini noodles and cook for about 2-3 minutes.
6. With a slotted spoon, transfer the zucchini noodles into a colander and immediately rinse under cold running water.
7. Drain the zucchini noodles well and transfer onto a large paper towel-lined plate to drain.
1. Divide the zucchini noodles onto serving plates evenly.
2. Remove the mushroom sauce from the heat and place over zucchini noodles evenly.
3. Serve immediately with the garnishing of parsley.

Nutritional Information per Serving:

Cal. 77 - Fats 4.6 g - Carbs 7.9 g - Prot. 3.4 g

EYE-CATCHING VEGGIES

Prep.: 51 min. | **Cook:** 20 min. | **Servings:** 4

Ingredients:

- ¼ C. butter
- 6 scallions, sliced
- 1 lb. fresh white mushrooms, sliced
- 1 C. tomatoes, crushed
- Salt and freshly ground black pepper, to taste
- 2 tbsp. feta cheese, crumbled

Directions:

1. In a large pan, melt the butter over medium-low heat and sauté the scallion for about 2 minutes.
2. Add the mushrooms and sauté for about 5-7 minutes.
3. Stir in the tomatoes and cook for about 8-10 minutes, stirring occasionally.
4. Stir in the salt and black pepper and remove from the heat.
5. Serve with the topping of feta.

Nutritional Information per Serving:

Cal. 160 - Fats 13.5 g - Carbs 7.4 g - Prot. 5.5 g

FAVORITE PUNJABI CURRY

Prep.: 15 min. | **Cook:** 35 min. | **Servings:** 3

Ingredients:

- 1 tbsp. olive oil
- ½ of small yellow onion, chopped finely
- 2 small garlic cloves, minced
- ½ tsp. fresh ginger root, minced
- 1 small Serrano pepper, seeded and minced
- 1 tsp. curry powder
- ¼ tsp. cayenne pepper

- 1 medium plum tomato, chopped finely
- 1 large eggplant, cubed
- Salt, to taste
- ¾ C. unsweetened coconut milk
- 1 tbsp. fresh parsley, chopped

Directions:

1. In a large skillet, heat the oil over medium heat and sauté the onion for about 6 minutes.
2. Add the garlic, ginger, Serrano pepper and spices and sauté for about 1 minute.
3. Add the tomato and cook for about 3 minutes, crushing with the back of a spoon.
4. Add the eggplant and salt and cook for about 1 minute, stirring occasionally.
5. Stir in the coconut milk and bring to a gentle boil.
6. Reduce the heat to medium-low and simmer, covered for about 20 minutes or until done completely.
7. Serve with the garnishing of the parsley.

Nutritional Information per Serving:

Cal. 105 - Fats 6.1 g - Carbs 12 g - Prot. 2.1 g

TRADITIONAL INDIAN CURRY

Prep.: 15 min. | **Cook:** 35 min. | **Servings:** 4

Ingredients:

- 3 tbsp. butter
- 7 oz. cottage cheese, cut into 2-inch cubes
- ½ head cauliflower, cut into small florets
- ½ C. water
- 1 C. fresh cream
- ½ C. Plain Greek yogurt
- 1-2 tbsp. curry paste
- 2 tbsp. fresh cilantro

Directions:

1. In a large skillet, melt half of the butter over medium heat and stir fry the cottage cheese cubes for about 4-5 minutes or until golden from all sides.
2. With a slotted spoon, transfer the cheese cubes onto a plate and set aside.
3. In the same pan, melt the remaining butter and cook the cauliflower for about 2-3 minutes, stirring frequently.
4. Stir in the water and cook, covered for about 4-5 minutes until all the liquid is absorbed.
5. Meanwhile, place the cream, yogurt and curry paste in a bowl and beat until smooth.
6. Stir the yogurt mixture into the frying pan and simmer for about 15-20 minutes, stirring occasionally.
7. Stir in the fried cheese cubes and cook for about 2 minutes or until heated through.
8. Garnish with fresh cilantro and serve hot.

Nutritional Information per Serving:

Cal. 215 - Fats 15.5 g - Carbs 8.1 g - Prot. 10 g

VINEGAR BRAISED CABBAGE

Prep.: 15 min. | **Cook:** 30 min. | **Servings:** 6

Ingredients:

- 2 tbsp. butter
- ½ head green cabbage, cut into ¼-inch slices
- ½ of yellow onion, sliced thinly
- 1 C. water
- 1 tbsp. Swerve
- 1 tbsp. organic apple cider vinegar
- 2 tsp. caraway seeds
- Salt, to taste

Directions:

1. In a large nonstick skillet, melt the butter over medium heat and sauté the cabbage, garlic and onion for about 5 minutes.
2. Add the remaining ingredients and stir to combine.
3. Immediately, reduce the heat to low and simmer for about 20-25 minutes.
4. Serve warm.

Nutritional Information per Serving:

Cal. 56 - Fats 4 g - Carbs 5 g - Prot. 1 g

GREEN VEGGIES CURRY

Prep.: 15 min. | **Cook:** 25 min. | **Servings:** 2

Ingredients:

- 3 tbsp. coconut oil, divided
- ¼ of small yellow onion, chopped
- 1 tsp. garlic, minced
- 1 tsp. fresh ginger, minced
- 1 C. broccoli florets
- 1 tbsp. red curry paste
- 2 C. fresh spinach, torn
- ½ C. coconut cream
- 2 tsp. low-sodium soy sauce
- 2 tsp. red boat fish sauce
- ¼ tsp. red pepper flakes, crushed
- 1 tsp. fresh parsley, chopped finely

Directions:

1. In a large skillet, melt 2 tbsp. of the coconut oil over medium-high heat and sauté the onion for about 3-4 minutes.
2. Add the garlic and ginger and sauté for about 1 minute.
3. Add the broccoli and stir to combine well.
4. Immediately, reduce the heat to medium-low and cook or about 1-2 minutes, stirring continuously.

5. Stir in the curry paste and cook for about 1 minute, stirring continuously.
6. Stir in the spinach and cook or about 2 minutes, stirring frequently.
7. Add the coconut cream and remaining coconut oil and stir until smooth.
8. Stir in the soy sauce, fish sauce, and red pepper flakes and simmer for about 5-10 minutes, stirring occasionally or until the curry's desired thickness.
9. Remove from the heat and serve hot with the topping of parsley.

Nutritional Information per Serving:

Cal. 324 - Fats 30.5 g - Carbs 11 g - Prot. 5.5 g

FUSS-FREE VEGGIES BAKE

Prep.: 15 min. | **Cook:** 20 min. | **Servings:** 6

Ingredients:

- 1 large zucchini, chopped
- 1 large yellow squash, chopped
- 1 medium green bell pepper, seeded and cubed
- 1 medium red bell pepper, seeded and cubed
- 1 yellow onion, sliced thinly
- 2 tbsp. olive oil
- 2 tsp. curry powder
- 1 tsp. ground cumin
- ½ tsp. paprika
- Salt and freshly ground black pepper, to taste
- ¼ C. homemade vegetable broth
- ¼ C. fresh cilantro, chopped

Directions:

1. Preheat the oven to 375°F.
2. Lightly, grease a large baking dish.
3. In a large bowl, add all the ingredients except cilantro and mix until well combined.
4. Transfer the vegetable mixture into the prepared baking dish and spread evenly.

5. Bake for about 15-20 minutes or until the desired doneness of the vegetables.
6. Remove from the oven and serve immediately with the garnishing of the cilantro.

Nutritional Information per Serving:

Cal. 83 - Fats 5.2 g - Carbs 9 g - Prot. 2.3 g

4 VEGGIES COMBO

Prep.: 20 min. | **Cook:** 12 min. | **Servings:** 5

Ingredients:

- 4 tbsp. butter
- ½ tsp. fresh ginger, minced
- 2 large garlic cloves, minced
- 1½ C. broccoli florets
- 1 C. carrot, peeled and julienned
- 1 tbsp. water
- 8 fresh shiitake mushrooms, sliced
- 1 C. canned water chestnuts, drained and sliced
- 1 tsp. arrowroot starch
- 3 tbsp. homemade vegetable broth
- 3 tbsp. low-sodium soy sauce
- ½ tsp. red pepper flakes, crushed
- Freshly ground black pepper, to taste
- 2 tsp. black sesame seeds, toasted

Directions:

1. In a large skillet, melt the butter over medium-high heat and sauté the ginger and garlic for about 1 minute.
2. Add the broccoli, carrot and water and cook for about 3-4 minutes.
3. Add the remaining vegetables and cook for about 2 minutes.
4. Meanwhile, in a bowl, add the arrowroot starch, broth and soy sauce and mix until well.
5. In the skillet, slowly add the broth mixture, stirring continuously until well combined.
6. Stir in the red pepper flakes and cook for about 3-4 minutes or until the vegetables' desired doneness, stirring continuously.
7. Stir in the black pepper and remove from the heat.
8. Serve hot with the topping of the sesame seeds.

Nutritional Information per Serving:

Cal. 118 - Fats 8.4 g - Carbs 8.4 g - Prot. 2.9 g

SNACK RECIPES

NO-CHURN ICE CREAM

Prep.: 10 min. | **Cook:** 0 min. | **Servings:** 3

Ingredients:

- Pinch salt
- 1 cup heavy whipping cream
- ¼ tsp xanthan gum
- 2 tbsp. zero calorie sweetener powder
- 1 tsp vanilla extract
- 1 tbsp. vodka

Directions:

1. You'll need an immersion blender and a jar that is pint sized with a wide mouth.
2. First, add the xanthan gum, heavy cream, vanilla extract, sweetener, vodka, and salt to a jar and mix.
3. Transfer the mixture to the immersion blender and, with the up-down motion, blend until you are left with a thick mixture.
4. This should take up to 2 minutes.
5. Put the mixture back in the jar, cover it, and place it in your freezer for 4 hours.
6. Remember to stir the cream mixture in 40 minutes' intervals.

Nutritional Information per Serving:

Cal. 291 - Fats 29.4 g - Carbs 3.2 g - Prot. 1.6 g

HIGH-PROTEIN EGG MUFFIN

Prep.: 10 min. | **Cook:** 20 min. | **Servings:** 6

Ingredients:

- 4 eggs

- 4 egg whites
- ½ cup organic unsweetened Greek yogurt or almond milk
- 1 cup chopped mushrooms
- 1 cup mix of chopped zucchini and chopped spinach
- ½ cup chopped onion

Directions:

1. Preheat oven to 385 degrees Fahrenheit.
2. Add onion to a pan coated with coconut oil and cook on medium heat until softened.
3. Add mushrooms, zucchini, and salt and pepper to taste.
4. Cook until softened.
5. Meanwhile, combine eggs, egg whites, and yogurt/almond milk in a bowl and beat thoroughly.
6. Add your cooked vegetables to your egg mixture.
7. Pour into muffin trays two-thirds of the way to allow for room to rise.
8. Bake for 20 minutes.

Nutritional Information per Serving:

Cal. 311 - Fats 19.4 g - Carbs 3.6 g - Prot. 8.9 g

CHEESECAKE CUPCAKES

Prep.: 10 min. | **Cook:** 15 min. | **Servings:** 12

Ingredients:

- 1 tsp vanilla extract
- ½ cup almond meal
- ¾ cup granulated no calorie sucralose sweetener

- ¼ cup melted butter
- 2 eggs
- 2 8 oz. pack softened cream cheese

Directions:

1. Preheat your oven to 350°F.
2. Also, prepare 12 muffin cups by lining them with paper liners.
3. Grab a bowl and put your butter and almond meal in it.
4. Using a spoon, take the almond meal mixture and put into the bottom of the muffin cup.
5. Press them down with the flat of the spoon to form a crust.
6. In a separate bowl, add vanilla extract, cream cheese, sucralose sweetener, and eggs.
7. Set an electric mixer to medium and combine the vanilla extract mixture until you get a smooth consistency.
8. Using a spoon, add this mixture to the top of the muffin cups.
9. Pop the muffin cups in the oven and bake until the center of the mixture is slightly set.
10. This should take no more than 17 minutes.
11. Now, you have your cupcakes.
12. Set them aside to cool.
13. When they are safe enough to hold again, put them in your refrigerator.
14. They should stay there 8 hours until the next day, when you can serve them.

Nutritional Information per Serving:

Cal. 209 - Fats 20 g - Carbs 3.5 g - Prot. 4.9 g

BROWNIES

Prep.: 10 min. | **Cook:** 30 min. | **Servings:** 12

Ingredients:

- ¼ tsp salt
- ¾ cup cocoa powder

- 1 tsp vanilla extract
- ½ tsp baking soda
- 1 ⅓ cups almond flour
- ⅔ cup coconut oil, separated
- 2 eggs
- ½ cup hot water
- 1 cup stevia sugar substitute

Directions:

1. Heat your oven to 350°F before you start.
2. Next, prepare an 8" pan by greasing it with coconut oil.
3. Get a medium bowl and throw your baking soda and cocoa powder into it.
4. Add the hot water and ⅓ cup coconut oil to the bowl.
5. Mix these ingredients properly until you have an even mixture.
6. Now, you can add what is left of your coconut oil, eggs, and stevia. Mix them some more.
7. Lastly, throw some salt, almond flour, and vanilla extract in the mix.
8. Stir the batter well until the ingredients are combined.
9. Turn this batter onto the pan you had prepared with coconut oil.
10. Next, pop the pan in the oven for about 35 minutes.
11. During this time, the top of the once-batter would have dried.
12. Take the pan out and let it cool.
13. Use a kitchen knife to cut 12 squares in the large brownie.

Nutritional Information per Serving:

Cal. 222 - Fats 20.5 g - Carbs 17.5 g - Prot. 5 g

CHOCOLATE PEANUT BUTTER CUPS

Prep.: 15 min. | **Cook:** 3 min. | **Servings:** 12

Ingredients:

- 1 oz. roasted peanuts, chopped and salted
- 1 cup coconut oil
- ¼ tsp kosher salt
- ½ cup natural peanut butter
- ¼ tsp vanilla extract
- 2 tbsp. heavy cream
- 1 tsp liquid stevia
- 1 tbsp. cocoa powder

Directions:

1. You'll need your stove at low heat for this recipe.
2. Place a saucepan on the heat and add coconut oil.
3. After about 5 minutes, add peanut butter, salt, heavy cream, cocoa powder, vanilla extract, and liquid stevia to the pan.
4. Stir till the peanut butter melts.
5. Get 12 silicone muffin molds and pour the peanut butter mixture in it.
6. Add the salted peanuts on top.
7. Transfer the muffin molds to a baking sheet and place the pan in your freezer.
8. Let it stay in the freezer for an hour, then unmold the cups.
9. Place the chocolate peanut cups in any airtight container.

Nutritional Information per Serving:

Cal. 246 - Fats 26 g - Carbs 3.3 g - Prot. 3.4 g

PEANUT BUTTER COOKIES

Prep.: 10 min. | **Cook:** 15 min. | **Servings:** 12

Ingredients:

- 1 tsp vanilla extract, sugar-free
- 1 cup peanut butter
- 1 egg
- ½ cup natural sweetener, low-calorie

Directions:

1. Preheat the oven to 350°F for this recipe.
2. Follow that by preparing a baking sheet. Line the sheet using parchment paper.
3. Into a bowl, add peanut butter, vanilla extract, sweetener, and egg.
4. Mix these ingredients well until you are left with dough.
5. Using your hands, mold the dough into balls.
6. These balls should be no more than 1 inch in size.
7. Place them on the baking sheet you had prepared and flatten them with a fork. You'll probably love the pattern that forms on the flattened dough.
8. Put the baking sheet in the oven and let the cookies bake for 15 minutes.
9. Afterwards, take the pan out of the oven and just let it sit.
10. After a minute of cooling, it should be safe for you to place on a wire rack to cool even further.

Nutritional Information per Serving:

Cal. 133 - Fats 11 g - Carbs 12 g - Prot. 5.9 g

LOW-CARB ALMOND COCONUT SANDIES

Prep.: 15 min. | **Cook:** 12 min. | **Servings:** 18

Ingredients:

- ⅓ tsp stevia powder
- 1 cup coconut, unsweetened
- 1 tsp Himalayan sea salt
- 1 cup almond meal
- 1 tbsp. vanilla extract
- ⅓ cup melted coconut oil
- 2 tbsp. water
- 1 egg white

Directions:

1. Your oven should be preheated to 325°F before you begin this dish. In addition to that, prepare a baking sheet by lining it with parchment paper.
2. Get a large bowl and put your Himalayan sea salt, unsweetened coconut, stevia powder, almond meal, vanilla extract, coconut oil, water, and egg white in it.
3. Stir this mixture properly.
4. Set the bowl aside for 10 minutes.
5. This is so that the unsweetened coconut will get considerably softer.
6. Mold the mixture into little balls. They should be small enough to fit on a tablespoon.
7. Place each ball on the prepared baking sheet. There should be some space between them.
8. Press down on the balls using a fork. Do this gently, as you don't want the edges to fall off.
9. Place the baking sheet in your oven and let the Sandies bake for about 15 minutes.
10. After letting the baking sheet cool for a minute, place it on a wire rack to get even cooler.

Nutritional Information per Serving:

Cal. 107 - Fats 10 g - Carbs 2.7 g - Prot. 1 g

CRÈME BRULÉE

Prep.: 10 min. | **Cook:** 34 min. | **Servings:** 4

Ingredients:

- 5 tbsp. separated natural sweetener, low calorie
- 4 egg yolks
- 2 cups heavy whipping cream
- 1 tsp vanilla extract

Directions:

1. Make sure that your oven is preheated to 325°F.
2. Also, get a bowl and put the vanilla extract and egg yolks in it. Use a whisk to mix them properly.
3. Set your stove to medium heat and put a saucepan on it.
4. Add 1 tbsp. of natural sweetener and heavy cream to the pan and mix using a whisk.
5. When you notice the mixture begin to simmer, take the pan down.
6. Get 4 ramekins and separate the mixture equally between them.
7. Place the ramekins in a glass baking dish and add hot water. The water should be an inch to the sides of the ramekins.
8. Place the glass baking dish at the oven center, and leave it there for 30 minutes. By this time, the Crème Brulée should have set.
9. Add 1 tbsp. natural sweetener on top of the Crème Brulée.
10. Here's the cool part: get a culinary torch and flame the sweetener until it turns a golden color and melts.

Nutritional Information per Serving:

Cal. 466 - Fats 48 g - Carbs 17 g - Prot. 5 g

CHOCOLATE FAT BOMB

Prep.: 10 min. | **Cook:** 0 min. | **Servings:** 10

Ingredients:

- 1.4 oz. pack instant chocolate pudding mix, sugar free
- 8 oz. pack cream cheese, softened
- Coconut oil to your preferred taste (suggested: ¾ cup)

Directions:

1. Into a medium bowl, add the chocolate pudding mix, cream cheese, and coconut oil. Use an electric mixer to combine these ingredients until they are smooth.
2. Place this mixture into a mold to form into mounds.
3. Cover these mounds with plastic wraps and keep in your refrigerator for about 30 minutes.
4. They should harden during this time.

Nutritional Information per Serving:

Cal. 231 - Fats 24.3 g - Carbs 3.5 g - Prot. 1.9 g

COCOA MUG CAKE

Prep.: 5 min. | **Cook:** 1 min. | **Servings:** 2

Ingredients:

- 2 tbsp. melted coconut oil
- 6 tbsp. almond flour
- 2 eggs
- 2 tbsp. cocoa powder, unsweetened
- Pinch salt
- 2 tsp natural sweetener, low-calorie
- ½ tsp baking powder

Directions:

1. Get a small bowl and add salt, almond flour, baking powder, cocoa powder, natural sweetener.
2. Into a second bowl, crack the eggs and beat with an electric mixer until you have a fluffy liquid. Next, add coconut oil and stir properly.
3. Pour this egg mixture into the previous bowl containing baking powder. Using a fork, whisk this mixture.
4. Prepare 2 mugs that are safe to go in a microwave by oiling them lightly.
5. Pour the mixture in your bowl into these cups.

6. Let there be some space at the top of the cups: at least, 1 inch. This is so that the cake will have room to rise without spilling over.
7. Set the microwave to high and place the cups inside it for 1 minute.
8. Take the cups out and check if the cakes have set and are done enough to serve. If not, put them back in the microwave.
9. Check the cakes every 10 seconds until you're satisfied that they are ready.
10. That is, the center of the cakes should not be runny.

Nutritional Information per Serving:

Cal. 338 - Fats 31 g - Carbs 8.6 g - Prot. 12 g

CHOCOLATE SHAKE

Prep.: 10 min. | **Cook:** 0 min. | **Servings:** 4

Ingredients:

- ¾ cup heavy (whipping) cream
- 4 ounces coconut milk
- 1 tablespoon Swerve natural sweetener
- ¼ teaspoon vanilla extract
- 2 tablespoons unsweetened cocoa powder

Directions:

1. Pour the cream into a medium cold metal bowl, and with your hand mixer and cold beaters, beat the cream just until it forms peaks.
2. Slowly pour in the coconut milk, and gently stir it into the cream.
3. Add the sweetener, vanilla, and cocoa powder, and beat until fully combined.
4. Pour into two tall glasses, and chill in the freezer for 1 hour before serving.
5. I usually stir the shakes twice during this time.

Nutritional Information per Serving:

Cal. 444 - Fats 47 g - Carbs 15 g - Prot. 4 g

Strawberry Shake

Prep.: 10 min. | **Cook:** 0 min. | **Servings:** 2

Ingredients:

- ¾ cup heavy (whipping) cream
- 1 tablespoon Swerve natural sweetener
- 6 ice cubes
- 2 ounces cream cheese, softened
- 6 strawberries, sliced

Directions:

1. Combine all your ingredients in your blender and process until smooth.
2. Pour into two tall glasses and serve.

Nutritional Information per Serving:

Cal. 407 - Fats 42 g - Carbs 13 g - Prot. 4 g

Latte Shake

Prep.: 10 min. | **Cook:** 0 min. | **Servings:** 2

Ingredients:

- 1 scoop unflavored collagen powder
- 1 tbsp. chia seeds
- 12 ounces cold brewed coffee
- 1 tbsp. MCT oil
- 1-2 tbsp. Swerve
- 1 cup unsweetened almond milk

Directions:

1. In a high-speed blender, add all the ingredients and pulse until smooth.
2. Transfer into 2 serving glasses and serve immediately.

Nutritional Information per Serving:

Cal. 144 - Fats 10 g - Carbs 4 g - Prot. 15 g

Vanilla Shake

Prep.: 10 min. | **Cook:** 0 min. | **Servings:** 2

Ingredients:

- 1 scoop unsweetened vanilla whey protein powder
- ½ cup heavy cream
- ¼ cup ice cubes
- 4-6 drops liquid stevia
- ½ tsp. organic vanilla extract
- 1½ cups unsweetened almond milk

Directions:

1. In a high-speed blender, put all the ingredients and pulse until creamy.
2. Pour the smoothie into two glasses and serve immediately.

Nutritional Information per Serving:

Cal. 190 - Fats 14.3 g - Carbs 3.4 g - Prot. 12.4 g

Garlic Parmesan Chicken Wings

Prep.: 10 min. | **Cook:** 3 hrs | **Servings:** 2

Ingredients:

- Chicken Wings (2 lbs.)
- Garlic (4 cloves, chopped)
- Coconut Aminos (1/2 cup)
- Fish Sauce (1 tbsp.)
- Sesame Oil (2 tbsp.)

Directions:

1. Put wings into a large bowl, drain or pat to dry.
2. In a small saucepan heat your ingredients, except wings.
3. Remove from flame and add sesame oil.
4. Pour mixture over wings and stir.
5. Cool and refrigerate overnight, you may stir occasionally as it marinates.
6. Remove wings from marinade and bake wings at 375°F until they are done.
7. Remove from heat and enjoy.

8. Add your favorite side dish or have as is.

Nutritional Information per Serving:

Cal. 738 - Fats 66 g - Carbs 4 g - Prot. 39 g

CATFISH BITES

Prep.: 12 min. | **Cook:** 16 min. | **Servings:** 6

Ingredients:

- 1-pound catfish fillet
- 1 teaspoon minced garlic
- 1 large egg
- ½ onion, diced
- 1 tablespoon butter, melted
- 1 teaspoon turmeric
- 1 teaspoon ground thyme
- 1 teaspoon ground coriander
- ¼ teaspoon ground nutmeg
- 1 teaspoon flax seeds

Directions:

1. Cut the catfish fillet into 6 bites.
2. Sprinkle the fish bites with the minced garlic.
3. Stir it.
4. Then add diced onion, turmeric, ground thyme, ground coriander, ground nutmeg, and flax seeds.
5. Mix the catfish bites gently.
6. Preheat the air fryer to 360°F.
7. Spray the catfish bites with the melted butter.
8. Then freeze them.
9. Put the catfish bites in the air fryer basket.
10. Cook the catfish bites for 16 minutes.
11. When the dish is cooked – chill it. Enjoy!

Nutritional Information per Serving:

Cal. 140 - Fats 8.7 g - Carbs 1.6 g - Prot. 13.1 g

SAVORY SALMON BITES

Prep.: 2 hrs. 5 min. | **Cook:** 0 min. | **Servings:** 12

Ingredients:

- Salmon trimmings (2 oz., smoked)
- Butter (2/3 cup, grass-fed, softened)
- Parsley (1 tbsp., chopped)
- Cheese (1 cup, mascarpone)
- Vinegar (1 tbsp., apple cider)
- salt (to taste)

Directions:

1. Use a fork to smash the cheese and add the remaining ingredients.
2. Form into small balls, and place on a tray lined with parchment paper.
3. Refrigerate for approximately 2 hours.
4. Serve.

Nutritional Information per Serving:

Cal. 117 - Fats 13 g - Carbs 1 g - Prot. 3 g

HERBED CHEESE FAT BOMBS

Prep.: 40 min. | **Cook:** 0 min. | **Servings:** 5

Ingredients:

- Cream cheese (3.5 oz., full fat)
- Olives (4 pitted, green, chopped)
- Herbs (2 tsp, dried)
- Parmesan cheese (5 tbsp., grated)
- Salt and black pepper (to taste)
- Butter (1/4 cup, unsalted)
- Tomatoes (4 pieces, drained, chopped, sun dried)
- Garlic (2 cloves, crushed)

Directions:

1. Blend together the butter and the cream cheese.
2. Transfer to a bowl.
3. Add the next four ingredients.

4. Season with salt and pepper, and mix.
5. Refrigerate for a minimum of 30 minutes.
6. Make 5 balls out of the mixture.
7. Roll each ball into the Parmesan cheese.
8. Serve.

Nutritional Information per Serving:

Cal. 164 - Fats 17.1 g - Carbs 2 g - Prot. 3.7 g

SAVORY FAT BOMBS

Prep.: 1 h | **Cook:** 5 min. | **Servings:** 6

Ingredients:

- 3.5 oz. cream cheese
- 1/4 cup (1.9 oz.) butter, cubed
- 2 large (2.1 oz.) slices of bacon
- 1 medium (0.5 oz.) spring onion, washed and chopped
- 1 clove garlic, crushed
- Salt to taste
- Black pepper, to taste

Directions:

1. Add your cream cheese to a bowl with your butter.
2. Leave uncovered to soften at room temperature.
3. While that softens, set your bacon in a skillet on medium heat and cook until crisp.
4. Allow it to cool then crumble into small pieces.
5. Add in your remaining ingredients to your cream cheese mixture and mix until fully combined.
6. Spoon small molds of your mixture onto a lined baking tray (about 2 tbsp. per mold).
7. Then place to set in the freezer for about 30 minutes.
8. Set your Air Fryer to preheat to 350°F.

9. Add to your Air Fryer basket with space in between each and set to air fry for 5 minutes.
10. Cool to room temperature.
11. When ready to serve, just spoon out 2 tablespoons (1.1 oz.) per serving.
12. Store in the fridge for up to 3 days.

Nutritional Information per Serving:

Cal. 108 - Fats 11 g - Carbs 0.6 g - Prot. 2 g

PORK BELLY FAT BOMBS

Prep.: 40 min. | **Cook:** 0 min. | **Servings:** 6

Ingredients:

- Bacon (3 slices, cut in half widthwise)
- Mayonnaise (1/4 cup)
- Horseradish (1 tbsp., fresh, grated)
- Lettuce (6 leaves, for serving)
- Pork belly (5.3 oz., cooked)
- Dijon mustard (1 tbsp.)
- Salt and pepper (to taste)

Directions:

1. Preheat the oven to 325°F.
2. Cook the bacon slices on a baking sheet for a minimum of 30 minutes in the oven. Let cool.
3. Crumble the bacon into a dish and set aside.
4. Shred the pork belly into a bowl and mix in the mustard, mayonnaise, and horseradish.
5. Season with salt and pepper.
6. Divide the mixture into 6 mounds.
7. Top with the crumbled bacon and serve on top of lettuce leaves.

Nutritional Information per Serving:

Cal. 263 - Fats 126 g - Carbs 0.5 g - Prot. 4 g

CHEESY PESTO FAT BOMBS

Prep.: 5 min. | **Cook:** 0 min. | **Servings:** 6

Ingredients:

- Cream cheese (1 cup, full fat)
- Parmesan cheese (1/2 cup, grated)
- Pesto (2 tbsp., basil)
- Olives (10, green, sliced)

Directions:

1. In a bowl, mix all the ingredients using a spatula, until well combined.
2. Serve as a dip with the cucumber (sliced) or other fresh vegetables.
3. You can also refrigerate for approximately 30 minutes.
4. Then create balls and roll into the Parmesan cheese.
5. Serve.

Nutritional Information per Serving:

Cal. 123 - Fats 13 g - Carbs 1.6 g - Prot. 4 g

DESSERT RECIPES

MUG CAKE

Prep.: 5 min. | **Cook:** 2 min. | **Servings:** 1

Ingredients:

- 1 egg, lightly beaten
- 1/8 tsp baking powder, gluten-free
- 2 tbsp. creamy peanut butter
- 1 tbsp. Swerve

Directions:

1. Add all ingredients into the microwave-safe mug and stir until well combined.
2. Place mug in microwave and microwave for 1-2 minutes.
3. Serve and luxuriate in.

Nutritional Information per Serving:

Cal. 257 - Fats 20.5 g - Carbs 9 g - Prot. 13 g

CHOCÓ FAT BOMBS

Prep.: 10 min. | **Cook:** 5 min. | **Servings:** 30

Ingredients:

- 3.5 oz. unsweetened dark chocolate
- 6 drops liquid stevia
- ¼ cup of coconut oil

Directions:

1. Add chocolate, oil, and sweetener in a microwave-safe bowl and microwave until chocolate is melted.
2. Pour chocolate mixture into the mold and place it within the refrigerator until set.
3. Serve and luxuriate in.

Nutritional Information per Serving:

Cal. 38 - Fats 3.6 g - Carbs 0.9 g - Prot. 0.4 g

DELICIOUS CHOCOLATE FROSTY

Prep.: 10 min. | **Cook:** 10 min. | **Servings:** 2

Ingredients:

- 1 ½ cups heavy whipping cream
- 2 ½ tbsp. lakanto monk fruit
- 1 tbsp. vanilla
- 2 tbsp. unsweetened cocoa powder

Directions:

1. Add all ingredients into the massive bowl.
2. Beat using the hand mixer until peaks form.
3. Scoop the mixture into the zip-lock bag and place it within the refrigerator for 45 minutes.
4. Remove a zip-lock bag from the refrigerator and cut the corner of the pack.
5. Squeeze frosty in serving bowls.
6. Serve chilled.

Nutritional Information per Serving:

Cal. 342 - Fats 34 g - Carbs 6.3 g - Prot. 2.9 g

STRAWBERRY MOUSSE

Prep.: 10 min. | **Cook:** 5 min. | **Servings:** 4

Ingredients:

- 1 cup heavy whipping cream
- 1 cup fresh strawberries, chopped
- 2 tbsp. Swerve

- 1 cup cream cheese

Directions:

1. Add heavy light whipping cream during a large bowl and beat until thickened using a hand mixer.
2. Add sweetener and cheese and beat well.
3. Add strawberries and fold well.
4. Pour in serving glasses and place within the refrigerator for 1-2 hours.
5. Serve chilled and luxuriate in.

Nutritional Information per Serving:

Cal. 320 - Fats 31 g - Carbs 6.2 g - Prot. 5 g

CHEESECAKE MOUSSE

Prep.: 10 min. | **Cook:** 5 min. | **Servings:** 6

Ingredients:

- 1 cup heavy whipping cream
- 1 tsp vanilla
- ¼ cup erythritol
- 8 oz. cream cheese, softened

Directions:

1. Add the cheese in a bowl and beat until smooth.
2. Add vanilla and sweetener and stir to mix.
3. In another bowl, beat heavy light whipping cream until stiff peaks form.
4. Fold topping into the cheese mixture and beat employing a hand mixer until fluffy.
5. Place in the refrigerator for two hours.
6. Pipe in serving glasses and serve chilled.

Nutritional Information per Serving:

Cal. 203 - Fats 20 g - Carbs 11 g - Prot. 3.3 g

DELICIOUS BERRY CHEESE DESSERT

Prep.: 10 min. | **Cook:** 10 min. | **Servings:** 8

Ingredients:

- 1 ½ lb. ricotta cheese
- 1 cup blackberries
- 1 cup blueberries
- 1 cup raspberries
- 1 ½ tsp vanilla
- ½ cup erythritol
- 1 tbsp. lemon zest
- ¼ cup heavy cream

Directions:

1. Add ricotta, vanilla, sweetener, and cream in a bowl and using a hand mixer, beat until smooth.
2. In four serving cups, place in layer alternating the ricotta mixture and ¼ cup of berries.
3. Serve and luxuriate in.

Nutritional Information per Serving:

Cal. 201 - Fats 12 g - Carbs 9 g - Prot. 10 g

CHOCÓ PEANUT BUTTER FUDGE

Prep.: 10 min. | **Cook:** 10 min. | **Servings:** 16

Ingredients:

- ½ cup peanut butter
- ½ tsp vanilla
- ¼ cup Swerve
- 2 ½ tbsp. unsweetened cocoa powder
- ¼ cup ghee

Directions:

1. Line a small baking dish with parchment paper and put aside.

2. Add ghee in a spread in microwave-safe bowl and microwave until ghee and spread are melted.
3. Add remaining ingredients and stir everything well and pour in prepared baking dish.
4. Place in refrigerator for 1 hour or until set.
5. Dig pieces and serve.

Nutritional Information per Serving:

Cal. 78 - Fats 7.4 g - Carbs 2 g - Prot. 2.2 g

RASPBERRY FAT BOMBS

Prep.: 5 min. | **Cook:** 5 min. | **Servings:** 8

Ingredients:

- ½ cup fresh raspberries
- 3 tbsp. Swerve
- 2 tbsp. coconut oil, melted
- 8 oz. cream cheese, softened

Directions:

1. Add all ingredients into the kitchen appliance and process until smooth.
2. Pour fat bomb mixture into the mini muffin mold and place it within the refrigerator for 45 minutes.
3. Serve and luxuriate in.

Nutritional Information per Serving:

Cal. 134 - Fats 13.3 g - Carbs 2.4 g - Prot. 2.2 g

QUICK LEMON MUG CAKE

Prep.: 5 min. | **Cook:** 2 min. | **Servings:** 1

Ingredients:

- 1 egg, lightly beaten
- ½ tsp lemon rind
- 1 tbsp. butter, melted
- 1 ½ tbsp. fresh lemon juice
- 2 tbsp. erythritol

- ¼ tsp baking powder, gluten-free
- ¼ cup almond flour

Directions:

1. During a small bowl, mix almond flour, leaven, and sweetener.
2. Add egg, juice, and melted butter in almond flour mixture and whisk until well combined.
3. Pour cake mixture into the microwave-safe mug and microwave for 90 seconds.
4. Serve and luxuriate in.

Nutritional Information per Serving:

Cal. 385 - Fats 32 g - Carbs 8 g - Prot. 13 g

SMOOTH & SILKY TIRAMISU MOUSSE

Prep.: 5 min. | **Cook:** 5 min. | **Servings:** 2

Ingredients:

- ½ cup mascarpone cheese
- 1 tbsp. erythritol
- 1 tsp unsweetened cocoa powder

Directions:

1. Add all ingredients into the blender and blend until smooth.
2. Pour blended mixture into the piping bag and pipe in serving glasses.
3. Place in refrigerator for 1 hour.
4. Serve chilled and luxuriate in.

Nutritional Information per Serving:

Cal. 110 - Fats 8 g - Carbs 2.4 g - Prot. 8 g

ALMOND MUG CAKE

Prep.: 8-10 min. | **Cook:** 10 min. | **Servings:** 1

Ingredients:

- 1/4 teaspoon baking powder

- 1/4 teaspoon vanilla extract
- 1 1/2 tablespoons cacao powder
- 1 egg, beaten
- 1/4 cup almond flour
- 1 teaspoon cinnamon powder
- 2 tablespoons stevia powder
- A pinch of salt

Directions:

1. Combine all ingredients within the bowl until well-combined. Add the combination during a heat-proof mug; cover with a foil.
2. Arrange Instant Pot over a dry platform in your kitchen. Open its top lid and switch it on.
3. Within the pot, pour water. Arrange a trivet or steamer basket inside that came with Instant Pot. Now place/arrange the mug over the trivet/basket.
4. Close the lid to make a locked chamber; confirm that the relief valve is in locking position.
5. Find and press "MANUAL" cooking function; timer to 10 minutes with default "HIGH" pressure mode.
6. Allow the pressure to create to cook the ingredients.
7. After cooking time is over, press the "CANCEL" setting. Find and press the "QPR" cooking function.
8. This setting is for quick release of inside pressure.
9. Slowly open the lid, calm down the mug, and serve warm.

Nutritional Information per Serving:

Cal. 138 - Fats 13 g - Carbs 7 g - Prot. 9 g

TAPIOCA KETO PUDDING

Prep.: 8-10 min. | **Cook:** 20 min. | **Servings:** 4

Ingredients:

- 1 tablespoon Erythritol

- 1 teaspoon chia seeds
- 1 tablespoon tapioca
- 1 tablespoon butter
- 2 cup heavy cream
- 1/4 cup raspberries or strawberries, mashed

Directions:

1. Arrange Instant Pot over a dry platform in your kitchen. Open its top lid and switch it on.
2. Find and press the "SAUTE" cooking function.
3. Within the pot, add the cream; cook (while stirring) for 4-5 minutes.
4. Add the tapioca and stir it well. Add the Erythritol and butter.
5. In a bowl, mix the chia seeds and berries.
6. Add the berry mix within the pot and stir well.
7. Close the lid to make a locked chamber; confirm that the relief valve is in locking position.
8. Find and press "MANUAL" cooking function; timer to fifteen minutes with default "HIGH" pressure mode.
9. Allow the pressure to create to cook the ingredients.
10. After cooking time is over, press the "CANCEL" setting. Find and press the "QPR" cooking function. This setting is for quick release of inside pressure.
11. Add in serving bowls, calm down, and place within the fridge for two hours.
12. Serve chilled.

Nutritional Information per Serving:

Cal. 246 - Fats 24 g - Carbs 10 g - Prot. 3 g

CREAM CHOCOLATE DELIGHT

Prep.: 8-10 min. | **Cook:** 15 min. | **Servings:** 4

Ingredients:

- 1 teaspoon orange zest
- 1 teaspoon stevia powder
- 2 heavy cream
- ¼ cup unsweetened dark chocolate, chopped
- 3 eggs
- 1 teaspoon vanilla extract
- ½ teaspoon salt

Directions:

1. Arrange Instant Pot over a dry platform in your kitchen. Open its top lid and switch it on.
2. Find and press the "SAUTE" cooking function.
3. Within the pot, add the cream, chopped chocolate, stevia powder, vanilla, orange peel, and salt; cook (while stirring) until the chocolate is melted.
4. Crack eggs within the pot, stirring constantly. Remove from the moment pot. Add the mixture to 4 mason jars with loose lids.
5. Within the pot, pour water. Arrange a trivet or steamer basket inside that came with Instant Pot. Now place/arrange the jars over the trivet/basket.
6. Close the lid to make a locked chamber; confirm that the relief valve is in locking position.
7. Find and press "MANUAL" cooking function; timer to 10 minutes with default "HIGH" pressure mode.
8. Allow the pressure to create to cook the ingredients.
9. After cooking time is over, press the "CANCEL" setting. Find and press the "QPR" cooking function. This setting is for quick release of inside pressure.
10. Slowly open the lid, calm down the jars, and chill within the fridge. Serve chilled.

Nutritional Information per Serving:

Cal. 254 - Fats 26 g - Carbs 5 g - Prot. 8 g

COCONUT KETO PUDDING

Prep.: 8-10 min. | **Cook:** 5 min. | **Servings:** 4

Ingredients:

- 3 tablespoons Stevia granular
- 1/2 teaspoon vanilla extract
- 1 2/3 cup coconut milk
- 3 egg yolks
- 1 tablespoon gelatin

Directions:

1. Arrange Instant Pot over a dry platform in your kitchen. Open its top lid and switch it on.
2. Add the coconut milk.
3. Close the lid to make a locked chamber; confirm that the relief valve is in locking position.
4. Find and press "MANUAL" cooking function; timer to five minutes with default "HIGH" pressure mode.
5. Allow the pressure to create to cook the ingredients.
6. After cooking time is over, press the "CANCEL" setting. Find and press the "QPR" cooking function. This setting is for quick release of inside pressure.
7. Place the coconut milk within the Instant Pot. Close the lid and confirm that the steam release valve is about to "Sealing."
8. Whisk in egg yolks and, therefore, the remainder of the ingredients.
9. Find and press the "SAUTE" cooking function. Cook until boiling the combination.

10. Add in serving bowls, calm down, and place within the fridge for two hours.

Serve chilled.

Nutritional Information per Serving:

Cal. 246 - Fats 27 g - Carbs 7 g - Prot. 4 g

CHOCOLATE LAVA CAKE

Prep.: 3 min. | **Cook:** 10 min. | **Servings:** 4

Ingredients:

- ½ cup raw unsweetened cocoa powder
- ¼ cup butter, melted
- 4 eggs
- ¼ cup sugar-free and gluten-free chocolate sauce
- ½ teaspoon ground cinnamon
- ½ teaspoon of sea salt
- 1 teaspoon pure vanilla extract
- ¼ cup raw stevia

Directions:

1. Pour 1 tablespoon of chocolate sauce into 4 cavities of an ice cube tray and freeze it.
2. Preheat oven to 350°F.
3. Prepare 4 ramekins by greasing with oil or butter.
4. Whisk together the cocoa powder, stevia, cinnamon, and sea salt in a small bowl.
5. Whisk in the eggs, one at a time.
6. Add the melted butter and vanilla extract. Stir until well combined.
7. Fill each prepared ramekin halfway with the mixture.
8. Remove the chocolate sauce from the freezer and place one in each of the ramekins.
9. Cover the chocolate with the remaining cake batter.

10. Bake for 13 to 14 minutes or until just set. Transfer from the oven to a wire rack and allow to cool for 5 minutes.
11. Carefully remove the cakes from the ramekins.
12. Enjoy your tasty and healthy chocolate lava cake by cutting into its molten center.

Nutritional Information per Serving:

Cal. 189 - Fats 17 g - Carbs 6 g - Prot. 8 g

DECADENT THREE-LAYERED CHOCOLATE CREAM CAKE

Prep.: 30 min. | **Cook:** 30 min. | **Servings:** 8

Ingredients:

- 4 ounces unsweetened chocolate
- ½ cup (1 stick) butter
- 1 ½ cups powdered sweetener, divided
- 3 eggs
- ½ cup + 8 tablespoons raw unsweetened cocoa powder
- 1 vanilla pod
- Pinch of sea salt
- 1 cup whipping cream
- Coconut whipped cream
- 1 can coconut milk, refrigerated overnight

Directions:

1. Preheat the oven to 325°F. Spray a little cooking oil into a pan smaller than 8 inches.
2. Combine the chocolate and butter in a double boiler and melt them together. Stir in ½ cup of sweetener and keep on stirring over low heat until everything is well combined. Remove from heat and let cool a little bit.
3. Separate the eggs, and beat the whites until stiff peaks form. Add ¼ cup of sweetener little by little.

4. Whisk the yolks together with another ¼ cup of sweetener. Add the chocolate mixture to the yolks and stir well. Mix in ½ cup cocoa, and then scrape the vanilla seeds from the pod and add to the mix and salt.

5. Fold in egg whites slowly to the chocolate mixture, but do not over mix.

6. Cook in the preheated oven for 1 hour or until a toothpick comes out clean. Let it cool completely and then remove from the pan.

Cream:

1. To prepare the 3 types of filling, beat the whipping cream for about 6-7 minutes until it gets very thick. Slowly add ½ cup of sweetener.

2. Divide the cream into halves and place one half in a bowl. Divide the remaining cream into halves again and place it in the other 2 separate bowls. You will have 3 bowls, one with ½ of the cream and two with ¼ of the cream.

3. Take a bowl with ¼ cream, add 1 tablespoon of cocoa powder and mix well. This will be the lightest-colored cream.

4. Add ½ the cream to the bowl, add 3 tablespoons of cocoa powder. Mix until well distributed. This will be the middle-colored cream.

5. Add 3–4 tablespoons of cocoa powder to the last bowl with ¼ cream. This will be the darkest cream.

Assembling:

1. Slice the cake horizontally in 3 equal slices using a very sharp knife.

2. Place the bottom part on a serving plate and cover with the middle-colored cream. Repeat with the second layer.

3. Top with the third cake piece and spread the light-colored cream on top, followed by the darkest cream.

4. Cut in 8 slices and enjoy.

Nutritional Information per Serving:

Cal. 304 - Fats 27 g - Carbs 11 g - Prot. 7g

INDIVIDUAL STRAWBERRY CHEESECAKES

Prep.: 10 min. | **Cook:** 0 min. | **Servings:** 4

Ingredients:

Crust

- ½ cup almond flour
- 3 tablespoons butter, melted (use coconut oil for a paleo version)
- ¼ cup sugar substitute (use pure Grade B maple syrup for a paleo version)

Filling

- 6 strawberries
- 3 tablespoons sugar substitute (use pure Grade B maple syrup for a paleo version)
- 8 ounces cream cheese (use full-fat unsweetened coconut cream for a paleo version)
- 1/3 cup sour cream (eliminate for a paleo version)
- ½ teaspoon pure vanilla extract
- 4 strawberries, quartered (for garnish)
- Fresh mint leaves (optional for garnish)

Directions:

1. To prepare the crust, place the almond flour, melted butter, and sugar substitute in a medium bowl and mix well to combine.

2. Divide the mixture evenly into 4 small serving bowls or ramekins, lightly pressing with your hands.

3. To prepare the filling, puree the strawberries in a food processor.

4. Add the sugar substitute, vanilla extract, cream cheese, and sour cream. Blend until smooth and creamy.

5. Spoon the mixture over the crust and chill for at least 1 hour.

Nutritional Information per Serving:

Cal. 489 - Fats 47 g - Carbs 12 g - Prot. 8 g

BROWNIE CHEESECAKE BARS

Prep.: 5 min. | **Cook:** 50 min. | **Servings:** 6

Ingredients:

Brownie layer:

- 2 ounces bittersweet chocolate, chopped
- ½ cup butter softened
- ⅓ cup raw unsweetened cocoa powder
- ½ cup almond flour
- 2 large eggs
- ½ cup sugar substitute
- ½ teaspoon pure vanilla extract
- ¼ teaspoon salt

Cheesecake layer

- 2 large eggs
- 16 ounces cream cheese, softened
- ⅓ cup sugar substitute
- ¼ cup heavy cream
- ½ teaspoon pure vanilla extract

Directions:

1. Preheat oven to 325°F.
2. Grease an 8x8 glass baking dish with butter or oil.
3. Melt the chocolate and butter together in a small saucepan over medium heat.
4. Stir until well combined.
5. Whisk the almond flour, cocoa powder, and salt together in a small bowl.
6. Whisk the eggs, sugar substitute, and vanilla extract in a large bowl until frothy.
7. Slowly whisk in the melted chocolate mixture.
8. Stir in the almond flour mixture and mix until smooth.

9. Pour into the prepared baking dish and bake for 20 minutes.
10. Transfer to a wire rack and allow to cool.
11. For the cheesecake layer, mix the cream cheese, eggs, sugar substitute, heavy cream, and vanilla extract with an electric mixer.
12. Reduce the oven heat to 300°F.
13. Pour the batter over the baked brownies and return to the oven for 40 to 45 minutes or until set.
14. Remove from the oven and cool in the fridge for at least 2 hours prior to serving.

Nutritional Information per Serving:

Cal. 566- Fats 54 g - Carbs 12 g - Prot. 13 g

RICH CHOCOLATE PUDDING

Prep.: 5 min. | **Cook:** 5 min. | **Servings:** 4

Ingredients:

- 2 cups coconut milk, canned
- ¼ cup raw unsweetened cocoa powder
- 1 tablespoon stevia
- 2 tablespoons gelatin
- 4 tablespoons water
- ½ cup heavy whipping cream, beaten to stiff peaks
- 1 ounce chopped bittersweet chocolate (optional for garnish)

Directions:

1. Heat the coconut milk, cocoa powder, and stevia in a small saucepan over medium heat.
2. Stir until the cocoa powder and stevia have dissolved.
3. Mix the gelatin with the water and add to the saucepan.
4. Stir until well combined.
5. Pour the mixture into 4 small ramekins or glasses.

6. Place the ramekins in the refrigerator for at least 1 hour.
7. Top with whipped cream, and chopped chocolate, if desired.

Nutritional Information per Serving:

Cal. 389 - Fats 37 g - Carbs 14 g - Prot. 8 g

FRESH STRAWBERRIES WITH COCONUT WHIP

Prep.: 5 min. | **Cook:** 3 min. | **Servings:** 4

Ingredients:

- 2 cans coconut cream, refrigerated
- 4 cups strawberries (can also use blueberries, blackberries, raspberries, or a combination)
- 1 ounce chopped unsweetened 70% or darker dark chocolate

Directions:

1. Scoop the solidified coconut cream (reserving the liquid in the bottom of the can for another use) into a large bowl and blend with a hand mixer on high for about 5 minutes or until stiff peaks form.
2. Slice the strawberries and arrange them in 4 small serving bowls.
3. Dollop the coconut whipped cream on top of the strawberries.
4. Garnish with chopped dark chocolate and additional berries.
5. Serve and enjoy!

Nutritional Information per Serving:

Cal. 342 - Fats 31 g - Carbs 15 g - Prot. 4 g

21-DAY MEAL PLAN

Day	Breakfast	Lunch	Snacks	Dinner	Dessert
1	Spinach, Mushroom, and Goat Cheese Frittata	Easy Keto Smoked Salmon Lunch Bowl	No-Churn Ice Cream	Crab Melt	Mug Cake
2	Cheesy Broccoli Muffins	Easy One-Pan Ground Beef and Green Beans	Cheesecake Cupcakes	Spinach Frittata	Chocó Fat Bombs
3	Berry Chocolate Breakfast Bowl	Easy Spinach and Bacon Salad	Brownies	Mushroom Omelet	Delicious Chocolate Frosty
4	Goat Cheese Frittata	Keto Smoked Salmon Filled Avocados	Garlic Parmesan Chicken Wings	Tuna Casserole	Strawberry Mousse
5	Zucchini Muffins	Summer Tuna Avocado Salad	Catfish Bites	Goat Cheese Frittata	Cheesecake Mousse
6	Spinach Omelet	Mushrooms & Goat Cheese Salad	Savory Salmon Bites	Meaty Salad	Delicious Berry Cheese Dessert
7	Easy Skillet Pancakes	Keto Bacon Sushi	Herbed Cheese Fat Bombs	Lemon Butter Fish	Chocó Peanut Butter Fudge
8	Quick Keto Blender Muffins	Keto Chicken Club Lettuce Wrap	Savory Fat Bombs	Lemon Garlic Shrimp Pasta	Raspberry Fat Bombs
9	Turmeric Chicken and Kale Salad with Food, Lemon and Honey	Keto Sheet Pan Chicken and Rainbow Veggies	Pork Belly Fat Bombs	One-Pan Tex Mex	Quick Lemon Mug Cake
10	Buckwheat Spaghetti with Chicken Cabbage and Savory Food Recipes in Mass Sauce	Shrimp Lettuce Wraps with Buffalo Sauce	Cheesy Pesto Fat Bombs	Spinach Artichoke-Stuffed Chicken Breasts	Smooth & Silky Tiramisu Mousse
11	Asian King Jumped Jamp	Poke Bowl with Salmon and Veggies	Chocolate Peanut Butter Cups	Chicken Parmesan	Almond Mug Cake
12	Keto Egg-Crust Pizza	Wrapped Bacon Cheeseburger	Peanut Butter Cookies	Sheet Pan Jalapeño Burgers	Tapioca Keto Pudding
13	Bacon Cheeseburger Waffles	Hearty Lunch Salad with Broccoli and Bacon	Low-Carb Almond Coconut Sandies	Grilled Herb Garlic Chicken	Cream Chocolate Delight

14	Sheet Pan Eggs with Ham and Pepper Jack	Fatty Burger Bombs	Crème Brulée	Blackened Salmon with Avocado Salsa	Coconut Keto Pudding
15	Classic Western Omelet	Avocado Taco	Chocolate Fat Bomb	Easy Cashew Chicken	Chocolate Lava Cake
16	Bacon Omelet	Chicken Quesadillas	Cocoa Mug Cake	Keto Creamy Chicken &Mushroom	Decadent Three-Layered Chocolate Cream Cake
17	Eggs in Avocado Cups	Salmon Sushi Rolls	Chocolate Shake	Chicken with Pablano Peppers &Cream	Individual Strawberry Cheesecakes
18	Crispy Chai Waffles	Mediterranean Salad with Grilled Chicken	Catfish Bites	Shrimp Sheet Pan Fajitas	Brownie Cheesecake Bars
19	Breakfast Roll-Ups	Cheese & Bacon Cauliflower Soup	Strawberry Shake	Chicken Bacon Ranch Casserole	Rich Chocolate Pudding
20	Frozen keto coffee	Shrimp and Avocado Lettuce Cups	Savory Salmon Bites	Spicy Lime Wings	Fresh Strawberries with Coconut Whip
21	Chocolate Pancakes	Salmon Wraps	Herbed Cheese Fat Bombs	Cheesy Meatball Bake	Raspberry Fat Bombs

21-DAY MEAL PAN FOR VEGETARIANS

Day	Breakfast	Lunch	Snacks	Dinner	Dessert
1	Cheese Crepes	Easy Keto Italian Plate	Cheesy Pesto Fat Bombs	Halloumi Time	Fresh Strawberries with Coconut Whip
2	Ricotta Pancakes	Fresh Broccoli and Dill Keto Salad	Herbed Cheese Fat Bombs	Poblano Peppers	Rich Chocolate Pudding
3	Yogurt Waffles	Low-Carb Broccoli Lemon Parmesan Soup	Vanilla Shake	Hash Browns	Brownie Cheesecake Bars
4	Broccoli Muffins	Prosciutto and Mozzarella Bomb	Latte Shake	Tomato Salad	Individual Strawberry Cheesecakes
5	Pumpkin Bread	Cole Slaw Keto Wrap	Strawberry Shake	Chili Lime Cod	Decadent Three-Layered Chocolate Cream Cake
6	Cheddar Scramble	Keto Broccoli Salad	Chocolate Shake	Keto Alfredo Zoodles	Chocolate Lava Cake
7	Sheet Pan Eggs with Veggies and Parmesan	Thai Cucumber Noodle Salad	Cocoa Mug Cake	Creamed Spinach	Coconut Keto Pudding
8	Almond Butter Muffins	Creamy Cauliflower Soup	Chocolate Fat Bomb	Parmesan-Crusted Cod	Cream Chocolate Delight
9	Crispy Chai Waffles	Creamy Tomato-Basil Soup	Low-Carb Almond Coconut Sandies	Cabbage Hash Browns	Tapioca Keto Pudding
10	Keto Breakfast Cheesecake	Spicy Cauliflower Soup	Peanut Butter Cookies	Cauliflower Hash Browns	Almond Mug Cake
11	Breakfast Roll-Ups	Black Soybean Soup	Chocolate Peanut Butter Cups	Cauliflower with Artichokes Pizza	Smooth & Silky Tiramisu Mousse
12	Frozen keto coffee	Avocado with Broccoli and Zucchini Salad	Brownies	Chili Cabbage Wedges	Quick Lemon Mug Cake
13	No-Bake Keto Power Bars	Cheesy Roasted Brussels Sprout Salad	Cheesecake Cupcakes	Cauliflower, Leeks and Broccoli	Raspberry Fat Bombs
14	Easy Skillet Pancakes	Zucchini Cauliflower Fritters	No-Churn Ice Cream	Roasted Green Beans with Parmesan	Chocó Peanut Butter Fudge

15	Quick Keto Blender Muffins	Curry Roasted Cauliflower	Chocolate Fat Bomb	Roasted Spicy Brussels Sprouts	Delicious Berry Cheese Dessert
16	Keto Everything Bagels	Roasted Brussels Sprouts with Pecans and Almond Butter	Cocoa Mug Cake	Sweet Creamy Cauliflower	Cheesecake Mousse
17	Creamy Porridge	Bell Peppers Soup	Strawberry Shake	Meat-Free Zoodles Stroganoff	Strawberry Mousse
18	Chocolate Pancakes	Spring Greens Soup	Herbed Cheese Fat Bombs	Eye-Catching Veggies	Delicious Chocolate Frosty
19	Lemon Poppy Seed Muffins	Alfalfa Sprouts Salad	Brownies	Favorite Punjabi Curry	Chocó Fat Bombs
20	Blueberry Bread	Loaded Baked Cauliflower	Peanut Butter Cookies	Vinegar Braised Cabbage	Mug Cake
21	Cheesy Broccoli Muffins	Radish Hash Browns	Latte Shake	Green Veggies Curry	Chocolate Lava Cake

CONCLUSION

Now that you are familiar with the Keto diet on many levels, you should feel confident in starting your Keto journey.

This diet plan will not hinder or limit you, so do your best to keep that in mind as you begin to make lifestyle changes and adjust your eating habits. When your body is stuffed with good fats and lots of protein, your body will transform and see these things as energy.

Before you know it, your body will have an automatically accessible reserve that you can use at any time. Whether you need a boost of energy first thing in the morning or a second wind to keep you going throughout the day, this will already be within you.

As you take care of yourself over the next few years, you can feel good knowing that the Keto diet aligns with the anti-aging lifestyle you seek. Not only does it keep you looking good and feeling younger, but it also acts as a preventative barrier from various ailments and conditions. The body tends to weaken as we age.

Yet, Keto helps keep a shield in front of it by giving you plenty of opportunities to burn energy and build muscle mass. Instead of taking the things you need to feel good, Keto only takes what you have in abundance.

This is how you will always end up feeling your best every day.

Arguably one of the best diets out there, Keto makes you feel good because you have so many options for meals! There's no shortage of delicious and filling meals that you can eat while you're on any Keto diet plan. You can even take this diet with you while you're eating out at a restaurant or a friend's house.

As long as you can remember the simple guidelines, you should have no problem staying on track with Keto. Cravings become almost non-existent as your body works to change the way it digests. Instead of relying on glucose in your bloodstream, your body changes focus. It starts using fat as soon as you reach the state of ketosis you are aiming for.

The Keto diet has been tried and tested for decades. It originated from a medical background to help patients with epilepsy.

Many successful studies align with the knowledge that Keto works. Whether you are trying to diet for a month or a year, both are equally healthy for you.

Good luck on your journey!

CPSIA information can be obtained
at www.ICGtesting.com
Printed in the USA
BVHW050035050521
606417BV00003B/832

9 781914 561023